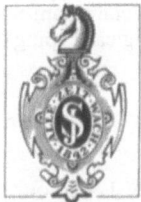

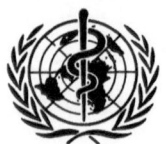 World Health Organization

The series *International Histological Classification of Tumours* consists of the following volumes. Each of these volumes – apart from volumes 1 and 2, which have already been revised – will appear in a revised edition within the next few years. Volumes of the current editions can be ordered through WHO, Distribution and Sales, Avenue Appia, CH-1211 Geneva 27.

1. Histological typing of lung tumours (1967, second edition 1981)
2. Histological typing of breast tumours (1968, second edition 1981)
3. Histological typing of soft tissue tumours (1969)
4. Histological typing of oral and oropharyngeal tumours (1971)
5. Histological typing of odontogenic tumours, jaw cysts, and allied lesions (1971)
6. Histological typing of bone tumours (1972)
8. Cytology of the female genital tract (1973)
9. Histological typing of ovarian tumours (1973)
10. Histological typing of urinary bladder tumours (1973)
12. Histological typing of skin tumours (1974)
13. Histological typing of female genital tract tumours (1975)
14. Histological and cytological typing of neoplastic diseases of haematopoietic and lymphoid tissues (1976)
16. Histological typing of testis tumours (1977)
17. Cytology of non-gynaecological sites (1977)
20. Histological typing of tumours of the liver, biliary tract and pancreas (1978)
21. Histological typing of tumours of the central nervous system (1979)
22. Histological typing of prostate tumours (1980)
23. Histological typing of endocrine tumours (1980)
24. Histological typing of tumours of the eye and its adnexa (1980)
25. Histological typing of kidney tumours (1981)

A coded compendium of the International Histological Classification of Tumours (1978).

The following volumes have already appeared in a revised edition with Springer-Verlag:
Histological Typing of Thyroid Tumours, 2nd edn. Hedinger/Williams/Sobin (1988)
Histological Typing of Intestinal Tumours, 2nd edn. Jass/Sobin (1989)
Histological Typing of Oesophageal and Gastric Tumours, 2nd edn. Watanabe/Jass/Sobin (1990)
Histological Typing of Tumours of the Gallbladder and Extrahepatic Bile Ducts, 2nd edn. Albores-Saavedra/Henson/Sobin (1991)
Histological Typing of Tumours of the Upper Respiratory Tract and Ear, 2nd edn. Shanmugaratnam/Sobin (1991)
Histological Typing of Salivary Gland Tumours, 2nd edn. Seifert/Sobin (1991)

A set of 124 colour slides (35 mm), corresponding to the photomicrographs in the book, is available from the American Registry of Pathology, 14th Street and Alaska Ave. NW, Washington, DC 20306, USA. For further information please see p. 113.

Histological Typing of Salivary Gland Tumours

G. Seifert

In Collaboration with L. H. Sobin
and Pathologists in 6 Countries

Second Edition

With 124 Figures

Springer-Verlag
Berlin Heidelberg New York
London Paris Tokyo
Hong Kong Barcelona
Budapest

G. Seifert
Institute of Pathology
University of Hamburg
Martinistrasse 52, UKE
W-2000 Hamburg 20, FRG

L. H. Sobin
Department of Gastrointestinal Pathology
and WHO Collaborating Centre
for the International Histological Classification of Tumours
Armed Forces Institute of Pathology
Washington, D. C., USA

In this series, colour illustrations will be limited in number in order to maintain a reasonable sales price.

The printing of the colour figures in this volume was made possible by a grant from the Jung-Stiftung für Wissenschaft und Forschung, Hamburg, Federal Republic of Germany.

First edition published by WHO in 1972 as No. 7 in the International Histological Classification of Tumours series

ISBN-13: 978-3-540-54031-1   e-ISBN-13: 978-3-642-84506-2
DOI: 10.1007/978-3-642-84506-2

Library of Congress Cataloging-in-Publication Data
Seifert, Gerhard, 1921– . Histological typing of salivary gland tumours / G. Seifert ; in collaboration with L. H. Sobin, and pathologists in 6 countries. – 2nd ed. p.   cm. – (International histological classification of tumours) Rev. ed. of Histological typing of salivary gland tumours / A. C. Thackray. 1972. Includes bibliographical references and index.
ISBN-13: 978-3-540-54031-1
1. Salivary glands–Tumours–Histopathology–Classification. I. Sobin, L. H. II. Thackray, A. C. Histological typing of salivary gland tumours. III. Title. IV. Series: International histological classification of tumours (Unnumbered) [DNLM: 1. Salivary Gland Neoplasms–classification. 2. Salivary Gland Neoplasms–pathology. WI 15 S459h] RC280.S3S45 1991 616.99'2316–dc20 DNLM/DLC for Library of Congress 91-4878 CIP

© Springer-Verlag Berlin Heidelberg 1991

21/3145-543210 – Printed on acid-free paper

Participants

Batsakis, J. G., Dr.
Division of Pathology, M. D. Anderson Hospital
and Tumor Institute, The University of Texas
System Cancer Center, Houston, Texas, USA

Brocheriou, C., Dr.
Laboratoire Central d'Anatomie et de Cytologie Pathologiques,
Hôpital Saint-Louis, Paris, France

Cardesa, A., Dr.
Catedrático de Anatomia Patológica, Facultad de Medicina,
Universidad de Barcelona, Barcelona, Spain

Dardick, I., Dr.
Departments of Pathology, Toronto Hospital and University
of Toronto, Toronto, Ontario, Canada

Ellis, G. L., Dr.
Department of Oral Pathology, Armed Forces Institute
of Pathology, Washington, DC, USA

Eveson, J. W., Dr.
Department of Oral Medicine, Surgery and Pathology,
Bristol Dental School and Hospital, University of Bristol,
Bristol, UK

Gusterson, B. A., Dr.
Department of Histopathology, The Institute of Cancer Research,
Royal Cancer Hospital, The Haddow Laboratories, Sutton, Surrey,
UK

VI   Participants

Seifert, G., Dr.
Institut für Pathologie der Universität Hamburg, Hamburg,
Federal Republic of Germany

Shanmugaratnam, K., Dr.
Department of Pathology, National University Hospital, Singapore, Republic of Singapore (WHO Collaborating Centre
for the Histological Classification of Upper Respiratory Tract
Tumours)

Sobin, L. H., Dr.
Department of Gastrointestinal Pathology, Armed Forces Institute
of Pathology, Washington, DC, USA (WHO Collaborating Centre
for the International Histological Classification of Tumours)

General Preface to the Series

Among the prerequisites for comparative studies of cancer are international agreement on histological criteria for the definition and classification of cancer types and a standardized nomenclature. An internationally agreed classification of tumours, acceptable alike to physicians, surgeons, radiologists, pathologists and statisticians, would enable cancer workers in all parts of the world to compare their findings and would facilitate collaboration among them.

In a report published in 1952,[1] a subcommittee of the World Health Organization (WHO) Expert Committee on Health Statistics discussed the general principles that should govern the statistical classification of tumours and agreed that, to ensure the necessary flexibility and ease of coding, three separate classifications were needed according to (1) anatomical site, (2) histological type, and (3) degree of malignancy. A classification according to anatomical site is available in the International Classification of Diseases.[2]

In 1956, the WHO Executive Board passed a resolution[3] requesting the Director-General to explore the possibility that WHO might organize centres in various parts of the world and arrange for the collection of human tissues and their histological classification. The main purpose of such centres would be to develop histological definitions of cancer types and to facilitate the wide adoption of a uniform nomenclature. The resolution was endorsed by the Tenth World Health Assembly in May 1957.[4]

---

[1] WHO (1952) WHO Technical Report Series. No. 53, 1952, p 45
[2] WHO (1977) Manual of the international statistical classification of diseases, injuries, and causes of death. 1975 version Geneva
[3] WHO (1956) WHO Official Records. No. 68, p 14 (resolution EB 17.R40)
[4] WHO (1957) WHO Official Records. No. 79, p 467 (resolution WHA 10.18)

Since 1958, WHO has established a number of centres concerned with this subject. The result of this endeavour has been the International Histological Classification of Tumours, a multivolumed series whose first edition was published between 1967 and 1981. The present revised second edition aims to update the classification, reflecting progress in diagnosis and the relevance of tumour types to clinical and epidemiological features.

General Preface to the Series

Among the prerequisites for comparative studies of cancer are international agreement on histological criteria for the definition and classification of cancer types and a standardized nomenclature. An internationally agreed classification of tumours, acceptable alike to physicians, surgeons, radiologists, pathologists and statisticians, would enable cancer workers in all parts of the world to compare their findings and would facilitate collaboration among them.

In a report published in 1952,[1] a subcommittee of the World Health Organization (WHO) Expert Committee on Health Statistics discussed the general principles that should govern the statistical classification of tumours and agreed that, to ensure the necessary flexibility and ease of coding, three separate classifications were needed according to (1) anatomical site, (2) histological type, and (3) degree of malignancy. A classification according to anatomical site is available in the International Classification of Diseases.[2]

In 1956, the WHO Executive Board passed a resolution[3] requesting the Director-General to explore the possibility that WHO might organize centres in various parts of the world and arrange for the collection of human tissues and their histological classification. The main purpose of such centres would be to develop histological definitions of cancer types and to facilitate the wide adoption of a uniform nomenclature. The resolution was endorsed by the Tenth World Health Assembly in May 1957.[4]

---

[1] WHO (1952) WHO Technical Report Series. No. 53, 1952, p 45
[2] WHO (1977) Manual of the international statistical classification of diseases, injuries, and causes of death. 1975 version Geneva
[3] WHO (1956) WHO Official Records. No. 68, p 14 (resolution EB 17.R40)
[4] WHO (1957) WHO Official Records. No. 79, p 467 (resolution WHA 10.18)

Since 1958, WHO has established a number of centres concerned with this subject. The result of this endeavour has been the International Histological Classification of Tumours, a multivolumed series whose first edition was published between 1967 and 1981. The present revised second edition aims to update the classification, reflecting progress in diagnosis and the relevance of tumour types to clinical and epidemiological features.

Preface to Histological Typing of Salivary Gland Tumours, Second Edition

The first edition of *Histological Typing of Salivary Gland Tumours*[1] was the result of a collaborative effort organized by WHO and carried out by the International Reference/Collaborating Centre for the Histological Classification of Salivary Gland Tumours at the Bland-Sutton Institute of Pathology, Middlesex Hospital, London, United Kingdom. The Centre was established in 1964, and the classification was published in 1972.

In order to keep the classification up to date, in 1987 a new group of participants was established, coordinated from the Institute of Pathology, University of Hamburg, Federal Republic of Germany. The participants are listed on pages V and VI. After histological slides and revision proposals were circulated among the participants, an informal meeting was held on the occasion of the XVIIth International Congress of the International Academy of Pathology in Dublin, Ireland, in September, 1988.

The preliminary result was a modified classification which was reported on in a Panel Discussion on the occasion of the XIIth European Congress of Pathology in Porto, Portugal, in September, 1989, and published in 1990.[2] After further communications, the present classification, definitions and explanatory notes were recommended for publication.

The histological classification of salivary gland tumours, which appears on pages 9–10, contains the morphology code numbers of

---

[1] Thackray AC, Sobin LH (1972) Histological Typing of Salivary Gland Tumours, Geneva, World Health Organization (International Histological Classification of Tumours, No. 7)

[2] Seifert G, Brocheriou C, Cardesa A, Eveson JW (1990) WHO International Histological Classification of Tumours. Tentative Histological Classification of Salivary Gland Tumours. Pathol Res Pract 186: 555–581

the International Classification of Diseases for Oncology (ICD-O)[3] and the Systematized Nomenclature of Medicine (SNOMED).[4]

It will, of course, be appreciated that the classification reflects the present state of knowledge, and modifications are almost certain to be needed as experience accumulates. Although the present classification has been adopted by the members of the group, it necessarily represents a view from which some pathologists may wish to dissent. It is nevertheless hoped that, in the interest of international cooperation, all pathologists will use the classification as put forward. Criticism and suggestions for its improvement would be welcomed; these should be sent to the World Health Organization, Geneva, Switzerland.

The publications in the series *International Histological Classification of Tumours* are not intended to serve as textbooks, but rather to promote the adoption of a uniform terminology that will facilitate communication among cancer workers. For this reason the literature references have intentionally been omitted and readers should refer to standard works for bibliographies.

---

[3] World Health Organization (1990) International Classification of Diseases for Oncology. Geneva
[4] College of American Pathologists (1982) Systematized Nomenclature of Medicine. Chicago

Contents

Introduction   1

Histological Classification of Salivary Gland Tumours   9

Definitions and Explanatory Notes 11

TNM Classification of Salivary Gland Tumours 39

Subject Index 49

Illustrations 51

Introduction

Knowledge of tumours of the salivary glands has advanced considerably in the two decades that have elapsed since work was started on the first edition of *Histological Typing of Salivary Gland Tumours*. A great deal of information has been collected about newly described tumour entities and the behaviour and prognosis of the previously classified tumours. Immunohistochemistry, cytophotometry, hybridization techniques, tissue culture and chromosomal analysis have increased our understanding of many tumours.

Histological Typing

Histological typing divides tumours of a given organ into different types according to their direction of differentiation. Although this may frequently indicate the underlying histogenesis of the tumour, it may be difficult or impossible to identify the cell of origin. Note is taken of the structure and function of cell types, as well as the overall growth pattern of the tumour, with the aim of matching these features to those of a normal tissue found in the same organ.

The principles of the second edition of the WHO *Histological Typing of Salivary Gland Tumours* are based on the following axioms:

- The classification is orientated to the routine work of the surgical pathologist. The inclusion of rare but clearly defined tumour entities should be helpful to surgical pathologists consulting with clinicians.
- The various types of carcinomas are distinguished not only by precise histopathological definitions, but also by differences in prognosis and treatment. For this reason, a continuous separate

listing of the various tumours is given rather than a histogenetic or other conceptual format.

Histological Grading

In contrast to the first edition of the WHO classification of salivary gland tumours, the term 'tumour' is here replaced by 'carcinoma' in two tumour entities: acinic cell carcinoma and mucoepidermoid carcinoma. All varieties of these lesions should be considered as potentially capable of metastasizing, regardless of their macroscopic or histological appearance.

In *acinic cell carcinoma* no histologic features or special growth patterns seem to have an obvious prognostic value. Prognosis is more dependant on local invasion and completeness of surgical removal. Therefore, no grading of acinic cell carcinoma is proposed.

Mucoepidermoid carcinomas can be categorized into low- and high-grade, and lesions so classified yield relatively good and bad prognostic groups with respect to local recurrence and metastatic ability. It should be remembered that these grades are part of a spectrum of histological features and though the features provide a good guide to behaviour, they have no absolute significance in individual cases. As with other malignant tumours, the adequacy of primary surgical excision is the major factor determining local recurrence, and taking this together with the other criteria a generally reliable prognostic assessment can be made.

In *adenoid cystic carcinoma* the histological characteristics are not as important prognostically as the anatomical site, size, surgical margins and clinical stage. All adenoid cystic carcinomas, regardless of their histological subtype, are biologically aggressive and can give rise to metastases many years after excision of the primary tumour.

Two other types of carcinomas, namely *polymorphous low grade adenocarcinoma* and *epithelial-myoepithelial carcinoma,* are associated with a usually good prognosis, whereas salivary duct carcinoma is characterized by a bad prognosis and resembles ductal carcinoma of the breast.

TNM Classification

The anatomical extent of disease is a major factor in assessing the prognosis of salivary gland carcinomas. The TNM classification, which appears on pages 39–47, provides a uniform system for recording, reporting and comparing data in regard to this.[1, 2]

Fine Needle Aspiration Biopsy

The overall type-specific diagnostic accuracy of fine needle aspiration biopsy for benign and malignant neoplasms of the salivary glands proceeding to surgery is high (over 80%). The accuracy is higher for benign than for malignant tumours. The sensitivity for the diagnosis of malignancy is about 80%, and the specifity is over 98%.

However, there are many problems and pitfalls; in particular, pleomorphic adenomas of variable histological patterns can be mistaken for several other types of tumour such as mucoepidermoid carcinoma or adenoid cystic carcinoma. Cystic changes can also lead to difficulties in interpretation.

For this reason, correct typing of the wide range of salivary gland neoplasms on the basis of cytological smears is difficult and requires extensive experience. Preoperative typing of tumours may be helpful in planning surgical treatment. It is important that the whole smear pattern be carefully assessed, including the quantity and the architectural grouping of the cells, the fine cytological detail such as chromatin pattern, nucleoli and cytoplasm, and the stromal components.

Air-dried smears stained with a Romanowsky stain give valuable information about stromal components, mucin secretion and cytoplasmic differentiation, whereas alcohol-fixed smears stained according to Papanicolaou are superior for the evaluation of nuclear chromatin and nucleoli, and reveal more detail within thick tissue fragments.

---

[1] Hermanek P, Sobin LH (eds) (1987) TNM Classification of Malignant Tumours, 4th edn. International Union Against Cancer. Springer-Verlag, Berlin Heidelberg New York

[2] Beahrs O, Henson DE, Hutter RVP, Myers M (eds) (1988) Manual for Staging of Cancer, 3rd edn. Lippincott, Philadelphia

The variability of histological patterns within the same tumour is an important problem in smears which can be only partly overcome by wide sampling. In ambiguous cases it is better to leave the differential diagnosis open rather than to risk a misleading report which could result in inappropriate surgery.

Cellular Differentiation

The cellular components of salivary gland tumours have important implications for clarifying diagnostic problems, for understanding histogenetic relationships, and for improving the classification of salivary gland tumours.

The *myoepithelial cells* have a hybrid epithelial and mesenchymal structure and functional phenotype. Neoplastically modified myoepithelial cells are generally accepted to be a significant component of salivary gland tumours, especially in pleomorphic adenoma, myoepithelioma, adenoid cystic carcinoma, epithelial-myoepithelial carcinoma and polymorphous low-grade adenocarcinoma. The light-microscopic features of myoepithelial cells in salivary gland tumours are described as spindle-shaped (myoid or fibroblast-like), plasmacytoid (hyaline), epithelial, and clear, usually glycogen-containing (see Sect. 1.2). These four types represent the cytomorphologic plasticity of the myoepithelial cells.

Clear cells are a feature of a wide variety of salivary gland neoplasms and the diagnosis of these tumours can be very difficult. The cytoplasmic clarity can be due to a number of factors including sparsity of organelles or storage of cytoplasmic contents such as glycogen, mucus, lipids and clear secretory granules, or it may be fixation artefact.

The majority of clear cell tumours are malignant. In benign tumours clear cells can be observed occasionally in pleomorphic adenoma (as clear myoepithelial cells), in clear cell oncocytoma (Sect. 1.5) and in sebaceous adenoma (Sect. 1.7). Primary carcinomas containing clear cells are mucoepidermoid carcinoma, acinic cell carcinoma, epithelial-myoepithelial carcinoma and sebaceous carcinoma. Foci of clear cells are common in mucoepidermoid carcinoma, and occasionally these cells are the main element of the tumour. Usually, however, examination of sufficient material will show areas of squamous differentiation. The cells of acinic cell carcinoma may become vacuolated or, more rarely, glass clear. It is exceptional for clear cells to form a significant proportion of the tumour. More typically there are adjacent granular or basophilic cells. Indeed, some consider clear cells in these tumours as fixation artifacts which reflect the length of time the specimen is left in formalin before processing. Epithelial-myoepithelial carcinoma forms ducts with an outer layer of clear cells. Their features are consistent with a myoepithelial origin. There is considerable variation in the proportion of small, dark duct lining cells to clear cells, and occasionally the latter are the predominant element, often forming sheets of cells rather than a duct-like structure.

The two metastatic clear cell tumours most likely to cause diagnostic difficulties are from renal or thyroid primaries. Occasionally, squamous cell carcinomas or melanomas contain clear cells. Histochemistry can help to distinguish metastatic clear cell carcinomas: for example, the clear cells of renal carcinoma contain abundant glycogen and lipid, while thyroid secondaries contain neither but are usually shown to contain thyroglobulin. However, sometimes it is not possible to exclude these secondary tumours by conventional microscopy, and further investigations such as CT scanning or intravenous urography may be necessary.

The salivary duct unit (intercalated, striated and excretory ducts) and reserve or stem cells give rise to all non-lymphoid, non-supporting tissue tumours of salivary glands. *Duct cells* are cellular elements of adenomas (pleomorphic adenoma, Warthin tumour, oncocytoma, canalicular adenoma, cystadenoma, ductal papilloma, etc.) and carcinomas (acinic cell carcinoma, mucoepidermoid carcinoma, epithelial-myoepithelial carcinoma, squamous cell carcinoma, adenocarcinoma, undifferentiated carcinoma, etc.).

Basal cells are the characteristic cell type of basal cell adenoma, basal cell adenocarcinoma and the solid subtype of adenoid cystic carcinoma. The basal cells are relatively isomorphic and show a prominent basal cell layer and the development of distinct basement membrane-like structures.

Value of Immunocytochemistry

Immunocytochemical techniques provide new data for the classification, functional differentiation and prognosis of salivary gland tumour pathology. Morphological tumour markers give information about cellular differentiation, proliferation and the functional status of tumours.

The three main types of epithelial cells of the salivary glands can be distinguished by tumour markers.

Acinic cells are characterized by the presence of amylase as well as cytokeratin, epithelial membrane antigen (EMA), lactoferrin, lysozyme, secretory component, carcinoembryonic antigen (CEA) and several blood group substances.

Ductal cells are immunoreactive with antibodies to cytokeratin, EMA, tissue peptide antigen (TPA), lactoferrin, lysozyme, secretory component, immunoglobulin A, lectin receptors, CEA and several blood group substances.

Myoepithelial cells are characterized by the absence of secretory products and the presence of actin, myosin and S-100 protein. A feature of modified myoepithelial cells is the double expression of both cytokeratin and vimentin. There appears to be a peculiar association of myoepithelial cells with basal membrane-associated substances, especially fibronectin.

In daily routine work the value of immunocytochemistry is limited with the exception of the following conditions:

– Amylase for the classification of the the clear cell variant of acinic cell carcinoma
– S-100 protein, actin or myosin for the identification of myoepithelial cells
– Cytokeratin for the distinction between undifferentiated carcinomas and malignant lymphomas or sarcomas
– CEA and thyroglobulin for the differential diagnosis of primary salivary gland adenocarcinoma and metastases of thyroid carcinoma

Cytophotometry

Cytochemical assessment of DNA content by means of scanning cytophotometry can be helpful in evaluation of salivary gland tumours.

Mucoepidermoid carcinomas and some types of adenocarcinoma show a strong correlation between biological behaviour and type of histogram, tumours with bad prognosis being identified by their 'atypical' histogram with aneuploidy.

Among adenoid cystic carcinomas, 'diploid' tumours have longer clinical courses than 'atypical' aneuploid ones.

Cytophotometry does not provide additional information for acinic cell carcinomas and epithelial-myoepithelial carcinomas, as virtually all have 'diploid' histograms which correlates with their low malignant potential.

Histological Classification of Salivary Gland Tumours

1   Adenomas

1.1	Pleomorphic adenoma	8940/0[a]
1.2	Myoepithelioma (Myoepithelial adenoma)	8982/0
1.3	Basal cell adenoma	8147/0
1.4	Warthin tumour (Adenolymphoma)	8561/0
1.5	Oncocytoma (Oncocytic adenoma)	8290/0
1.6	Canalicular adenoma	
1.7	Sebaceous adenoma	8410/0
1.8	Ductal papilloma	8503/0
1.8.1	Inverted ductal papilloma	8053/0
1.8.2	Intraductal papilloma	8503/0
1.8.3	Sialadenoma papilliferum	8260/0
1.9	Cystadenoma	8440/0
1.9.1	Papillary cystadenoma	8450/0
1.9.2	Mucinous cystadenoma	8470/0

2   Carcinomas

2.1	Acinic cell carcinoma	8550/3
2.2	Mucoepidermoid carcinoma	8430/3
2.3	Adenoid cystic carcinoma	8200/3
2.4	Polymorphous low grade adenocarcinoma (Terminal duct adenocarcinoma)	
2.5	Epithelial-myoepithelial carcinoma	8562/3
2.6	Basal cell adenocarcinoma	8147/3
2.7	Sebaceous carcinoma	8410/3

---

[a] Morphology code of the International Classification of Diseases for Oncology (ICD-O) and the Systematized Nomenclature of Medicine (SNOMED)

2.8	Papillary cystadenocarcinoma	8450/3
2.9	Mucinous adenocarcinoma	8480/3
2.10	Oncocytic carcinoma	8290/3
2.11	Salivary duct carcinoma	8500/3
2.12	Adenocarcinoma	8140/3
2.13	Malignant myoepithelioma (Myoepithelial carcinoma)	8982/3
2.14	Carcinoma in pleomorphic adenoma (Malignant mixed tumour)	8941/3
2.15	Squamous cell carcinoma	8070/3
2.16	Small cell carcinoma	8041/3
2.17	Undifferentiated carcinoma	8020/3
2.18	Other carcinomas	

3   Non-epithelial Tumours

4   Malignant Lymphomas

5   Secondary Tumours

6   Unclassified Tumours

7   Tumour-like Lesions

7.1	Sialadenosis	71000
7.2	Oncocytosis	73050
7.3	Necrotizing sialometaplasia (Salivary gland infarction)	73220
7.4	Benign lymphoepithelial lesion	72240
7.5	Salivary gland cysts	33400
7.6	Chronic sclerosing sialadenitis of submandibular gland (Küttner tumour)	45000
7.7	Cystic lymphoid hyperplasia in AIDS	

Definitions and Explanatory Notes

1 Adenomas

1.1 Pleomorphic Adenoma (Figs. 1–5)

A tumour of variable capsulation characterized microscopically by architectural rather than cellular pleomorphism. Epithelial and modified myoepithelial elements intermingle with tissue of mucoid, myxoid or chondroid appearance. The epithelial and myoepithelial components form ducts, strands, sheets or structures resembling a swarm of bees. Squamous metaplasia is found in about 25% of pleomorphic adenomas.

The modified myoepithelial cells are usually polygonal in the solid sheets, or they may be spindle-shaped. They are eosinophilic or clear. The arrangement of modified myoepithelial cells in sheets or surrounding duct-like structures is an essential element for diagnosing pleomorphic adenoma, as is the lack of a clear-cut boundary between the epithelial elements and the stroma (in contrast to myoepithelioma, see Sect. 1.2). The mucoid, myxoid, chondroid or hyaline material is generally interpreted as being the product of the myoepithelial cells.

Attempts have been made to subclassify pleomorphic adenomas on the basis of the differentiation of the epithelial cells and the proportion and differentiation of the stroma. It has been suggested that cell-rich variants have a higher risk of malignant transformation and that cell-poor tumours have a higher risk of recurrence. However, the range of histological appearances within an individual tumour can be extremely variable, which makes subclassification difficult.

The significant risk of recurrence, particularly in the days before parotidectomy became standard treatment, is probably due to a variety of reasons, mainly related to the anatomical features of the tumour. Some pleomorphic adenomas are diffluent and easily rupture during removal. Although they tend to be discrete, they can bulge through the capsule or extend into the surrounding tissue. The former is variable in thickness and may be incomplete or absent. In addition, pleomorphic adenomas have a tendency to show intracapsular invasion, and a plane of weakness between the capsule and the main tumour mass. It is also possible that the tumour cells, like those of chondroid neoplasms, have low biological requirements and therefore readily survive when material is inadvertently spilt into the wound.

Exceptionally rarely, an apparently typical pleomorphic adenoma may give rise to distant metastases with a microscopical appearance similar to that of the primary (see Sect. 2.14).

1.2 Myoepithelioma (Myoepithelial Adenoma) (Figs. 6, 7)

A rare tumour of myoepithelial cells; several growth patterns occur: solid, myxoid and reticular.

The cellular components are spindle-shaped, plasmacytoid (hyaline), epithelioid and clear cells or combinations of these. Most myoepitheliomas have a solid growth pattern and cells with hyaline cytoplasm, eccentric nuclei and discrete nucleoli. The reticular type shows an intricate, sieve-like pattern with narrow anastomosing cords of spindle cells ramifying through a mucoid, relatively acellular stroma.

The immunohistochemical demonstration of S-100 protein, actin or myosin is of practical value in defining myoepithelial cells. There is a close relationship between myoepithelioma and pleomorphic adenoma as both contain myoepithelial cells. Unlike pleomorphic adenoma, myoepithelioma does not show ductal differentiation but does exhibit sharp demarcation of the cellular cords from the myxoid-vascular stroma. The distinction is important because myoepithelioma is characterized by more aggressive growth than pleomorphic adenoma and occasionally by transformation to malignancy (see Sect. 2.13). The parotid and palate are the sites of predilection. Myoepitheliomas are rare tumours (less than 1% of all salivary gland tumours).

1.3 Basal Cell Adenoma (Figs. 8–11)

A tumour of isomorphic basaloid cells with a prominent basal cell layer, a distinct basement membrane-like structure and no mucoid stromal component as in pleomorphic adenomas. Four cellular patterns occur: solid, trabecular, tubular and membranous.

The *solid variant* consists of uniform-appearing, generally small cells. These are arranged in relatively large compact aggregates in which the outer layer often is palisaded. In addition, intercellular deposits occur, as does focal squamous differentiation and basisquamous whorls in the globular ends of epithelial islands.

The *trabecular* and *tubular variants* have a major component of basaloid cells arranged in narrow, anastomosing bands or on the outer aspect of ductal structures. Combinations of both growth patterns to varying degrees are common. Even in the trabecular form glandular differentiation, i. e. an inner layer of slightly larger luminal cells, may be evident.

The *membranous variant (dermal anlage type)* is characterized by palisading of peripheral cells and an excessive hyaline basal membrane. In initial stages, focal ductal hyperplasia with proliferation of basal cells and microadenomas can be observed. As a result, multifocal and multinodular tumours develop in the parotid gland and also in the submandibular gland in the same patient.

There is a characteristic association with dermal cylindroma (turban tumour), trichoepithelioma or eccrine spiradenoma of the scalp. This combination represents a peculiar inherited tumour diathesis involving neoplasms of presumed ductal origin.

Basal cell adenoma can transform to basal cell adenocarcinoma (Sect. 2.6).

The frequency of basal cell adenoma is 1%–2% of all salivary gland tumours, with an age peak in the 7th decade of life. The main locations are the parotid gland (70%) and the minor salivary glands of the upper lip (20%).

1.4 Warthin Tumour (Adenolymphoma) (Figs. 12–16)

A tumour composed of glandular and often cystic structures, sometimes with a papillary cystic arrangement, lined by characteristic eosinophilic epithelium. The stroma contains a variable amount of lymphoid tissue with follicles.

The epithelium is double-layered, the inner cells being high columnar with abundant finely granular acidophilic cytoplasm. Rarely, there may be goblet cells with mucous secretion or groups of sebaceous cells. The amount of lymphoid tissue is variable.

A rare subtype, variously termed metaplastic, infected or infarcted Warthin tumour, has much of the original oncocytic epithelium replaced by squamous cells, which can make the tumours resemble a ruptured epidermoid or lymphoepithelial cyst. Extensive epithelioid granuloma formation in the stroma can resemble tuberculosis. Classification into stroma-rich and stroma-poor subtypes is possible but is without prognostic value.

With rare exceptions this tumour arises only in the parotid gland. The main localization at the lower pole of the parotid gland supports development from parenchymal inclusions in the parotid lymph nodes.

The tumour is found predominantly in males. The age peak is in the 6th and 7th decades. The term Warthin tumour is preferred over the earlier designation 'adenolymphoma' which could be confused with malignant lymphoma. The term 'papillary cystadenoma lymphomatosum' is accurate but cumbersome.

1.5 Oncocytoma (Oncocytic Adenoma) (Figs. 17–19)

A rare tumour composed of a well demarcated mass of polyhedral eosinophilic cells with small, dark nuclei. It has a solid, trabecular or tubular pattern and frequently contains both light and dark cells.

The tumour is usually surrounded by a thin capsule which may be incomplete. It occurs predominantly in the parotid gland of older adults. The intensely eosinophilic granular cytoplasm is due to large numbers of mitochondria. Cytoplasmic staining of mitochondria with phosphotungstic acid-haematoxylin (PTAH) can be helpful for the diagnosis of oncocytes. Oncocytoma may originate from multifocal oncocytic hyperplasia, which acquires the autonomous growth of a benign neoplasm.

Multifocal oncocytic adenomatous hyperplasia (see Sect. 7.2) consists of non-encapsulated nodules of oncocytic or clear cells in the parotid gland. The nodules have a lobular distribution and normal acinar tissue may be included at the periphery. The presence of satellite foci may give the false impression that the lesion is an invasive neoplasm.

Clear cell oncocytoma is a rare variant which consists of a circumscribed mass of polyhedral cells with clear cytoplasm and small, dark, eccentrically located nuclei. The cells may be arranged in an organoid pattern separated by thin, fibrous septa. Staining with PTAH may show the granular positivity of mitochondria. Variable amounts of glycogen may be detected with periodic acid-Schiff staining, but mucous stains are negative. The clear cell oncocytoma is probably the only benign clear cell salivary gland tumour.

Diffuse oncocytosis is discussed in Sect. 7.2.

1.6 Canalicular Adenoma (Figs. 20, 21)

A tumour of columnar epithelial cells which are arranged in anastomosing bilayered strands that form a beading pattern. The stroma is loose, highly vascular and not fibrous.

The tumour is localized to the upper lip in 90% of cases and in almost all cases occurs in patients over 50 years of age.

The tumour is distinguished from the trabecular type of basal cell adenoma which has a fibrous rather than a loose, vascularized stroma. There is no association with dermal cylindroma.

1.7 Sebaceous Adenoma (Figs. 22, 23)

A rare tumour consisting of irregular nests of sebaceous cells without cellular atypia. The tumour is typically well circumscribed and cystic.

Sebaceous lymphadenoma is a rare but distinctive variant of sebaceous adenoma with groups of well-differentiated sebaceous cells arranged in a glandular configuration with associated ducts of variable size, lying in a stroma of lymphocytes, with or without follicles.

The similarity to Warthin tumour suggests a common mode of development, possibly from salivary duct inclusions within a parotid lymph node, with metaplasia of the epithelium to sebaceous rather than oncocytic cells.

Unilocular cystic sebaceous lymphadenoma is a lymphoepithelial cyst with sebaceous differentiation. Sebaceous differentiation, the result of metaplasia of the duct lining cells, is not uncommon in salivary glands, particularly the parotid gland, but sebaceous neoplasms are rare.

1.8 Ductal Papilloma (Figs. 24–28)

1.8.1 Inverted Ductal Papilloma

An extremely rare but distinct tumour that arises from the excretory ducts and resembles the inverted papilloma of the nasal and paranasal sinuses, both in growth pattern and cytologically.

The squamous epithelial cells extend into the surrounding connective tissue. The proliferating tissue can be seen in continuity with normal ducts. Mucous cells and microcysts may be present in the epithelium. This tumour occurs predominantly in the minor salivary glands.

1.8.2 Intraductal Papilloma

A very rare solitary tumour of the excretory ducts of minor salivary glands. The tumour consists of papillary intraductal projections with connective tissue cores that extend into widely dilated ducts or cystic spaces. The ingrowths are lined by one or two layers of benign, cuboidal or squamous epithelium.

There are similarities to the solitary intraductal papilloma of the breast.

1.8.3 Sialadenoma Papilliferum

An exophytic growth mainly in the palate with multiple papillary surface fronds and deeper duct-like structures which may be in continuity with the surface.

The duct-like structures typically have a distinct, double layer and may be thrown into small papillary projections. Among the papillary fronds squamous epithelium can be observed. Recurrence is uncommon. The tumour resembles the cutaneous syringocystadenoma papilliferum and also bears similarities to Warthin tumour.

1.9 Cystadenoma (Figs. 29–31)

1.9.1 Papillary Cystadenoma

A tumour that closely resembles Warthin tumour but without the lymphoid elements.

Most cases have been described in the larynx, and occurrence in the salivary glands is rare. In contrast to the intraductal papilloma, the papillary cystadenoma is multicystic with multiple papillary projections and a greater variety of epithelial lining cells.

1.9.2 Mucinous Cystadenoma

A circumscribed tumour with cystic spaces lined by mucus-producing cells or goblet cells but no cellular atypia or invasive growth.

Great care is needed to differentiate these benign tumours from their more common malignant counterpart, mucinous adenocarcinoma (Sect. 2.9).

2 Carcinomas

2.1 Acinic Cell Carcinoma (Figs. 32–39)

A malignant epithelial neoplasm that demonstrates some cytological differentiation toward acinar cells.

Gross examination of parotidectomy specimens typically demonstrates that primary (first occurrence) acinic cell carcinomas are mononodular; however, multinodularity is not infrequent. Some tumours may appear to be encapsulated, but microscopically this is usually found to be incomplete. They may be solid or cystic.

Acinic cell carcinoma has a wide spectrum of *histopathological features*. The morphological growth patterns can be described as *solid, microcystic, papillary-cystic,* and *follicular.* The individual cell characteristics can be categorized as acinar, intercalated duct-like, vacuolated, clear and non-specific glandular. Any or all of these morphologic patterns and cell types may be seen in an individual tumour, and indeed commonly are. In fact, it has been the occurrence of well-differentiated acinar cells in association with the other cell types and morphologic patterns that has enabled us to define the broad spectrum of acinic cell carcinoma.

Acinar cells are usually identified by their relatively large size, round to polygonal shape, basophilic to amphophilic cytoplasm, and dark staining cytoplasmic granules similar to those of normal parenchymal acinar cells. Periodic acid-Schiff stain will highlight the cytoplasmic granules. Some of these cells can be found in nearly all acinic

cell carcinomas. The intercalated duct-like cells are smaller than acinar cells and cuboidal in shape. Their cytoplasm is amphophilic to
acidophilic. The nuclei are centrally placed and about the same size
as the acinar cells, so that the nucleus-to-cytoplasm ratio is increased. Often these cells surround small lumina. The vacuolated
cells are peculiar and seem unique to acinic cell carcinomas among
salivary gland neoplasms. These cells are typically about the size of
the well-differentiated acinar cells, although some appear to be distended by the cytoplasmic vacuoles. The cytoplasmic compartment
is punctuated by clear vacuoles that occupy most of the cytoplasm.
There may be several vacuoles or a single large vacuole. Stains for lipids and glycogen demonstrate no material in the vacuoles, but there
may be some mucopolysaccharides. The vacuolated cells are most
evident in the microcystic and papillary cystic growth patterns. Clear
cells occur in only a small number of acinic cell carcinomas and
usually only compose a small part of the tumour. They have the
shape and morphology of acinar or intercalated duct-like cells that
have lost their cytoplasmic staining. The non-specific glandular cells
are defined by the absence of features characteristic of the other
four cell types. They usually form a syncytium of cells with indistinct
cell boundaries and amphophilic cytoplasm. The nuclei are typically
larger, more vesicular, and more pleomorphic than those of the
other cell types.

A *solid growth pattern* is the most easily recognized morphological variant of acinic cell carcinoma because it usually contains large
numbers of well-differentiated acinar cells and most closely resembles the normal parotid gland parenchyma. In the solid pattern the
tumour is composed of sheets of tumour cells that frequently have
an organoid configuration.

The *microcystic pattern* shows numerous small cystic spaces
which are about three to ten times the size of acinar cells. Well-differentiated acinar cells are still quite frequent and may even be
dominant in this pattern, but vacuolated and intercalated duct-like
cells can also be prominent. It appears that the microcystic spaces
may result from the coalescence of intracellular vacuoles of ruptured
cells. Proteinaceous or mucinous material may pool in the microcystic spaces.

The *papillary cystic growth pattern* is characterized by one or
more cystic structures that contain proliferations of epithelium. The
cysts may be small with a few folds of lining epithelium, or quite
large with long stalks, fronds, or masses of glandular epithelium

within the lumens. Some of the epithelial projections will have thin fibrovascular cores, while others appear to be masses of epithelium without apparent supporting stroma. Intercalated duct-like and non-specific glandular cells usually predominate, although vacuolated cells are often numerous and acinar cells can be seen. The apical portion of many of the lumen-lining cells bulges into the lumen and produces a tombstone or hobnail-like conformation. The papillary cystic pattern occurs less frequently than the microcystic or solid growth patterns.

The *follicular pattern* of acinic cell carcinoma is the least often encountered. This pattern has a definite thyroid-like appearance. Variable sized, ovoid to round cystic spaces are lined by cuboidal to low columnar epithelial cells. Many of the cystic spaces contain an eosinophilic proteinaceous material that simulates the appearance of colloid. The intercystic areas are usually occupied by epithelial cells that are mostly non-specific glandular cells, with some vacuolated and acinar type cells.

One of the curious features of acinic cell carcinoma is the frequent association with a lymphoid infiltrate in the supporting stroma.

Acinic cell carcinomas are regarded as low-grade malignancies. Microscopic examination demonstrates most of these tumours to be infiltrative. Neither any of the four histological growth patterns nor predominance of any one of the five cell types has been found to be reliably predictive of a more favourable or worse clinical course.

While not common, acinic cell carcinoma is one of the more frequently encountered malignant tumours of the parotid gland. Published large series of salivary gland tumours have shown the frequency of acinic cell carcinoma to range from 1.4% to 20.0% of malignant parotid gland tumors.

The parotid gland is the predominant site of occurrence (81%) of acinic cell carcinoma. Only about 4% occur in the submandibular gland, and 13% develop in the minor salivary glands. The buccal mucosa, upper lip, and palate, in that order, are the most frequent minor salivary gland sites of occurrence. A predominance of female patients has been observed. This tumour occurs in patients of all age groups, including children; the mean age is in the 5th decade of life.

2.2 Mucoepidermoid Carcinoma (Figs. 40–48)

A tumour characterized by the presence of squamous cells, mucus-producing cells, and cells of intermediate type.

The gross appearance varies with grade, but most tumours are poorly circumscribed and usually show cyst formation. The cysts contain clear or straw-coloured, mucoid fluid and there may be intracystic haemorrhage. The proportion of the different cell types and their architectural configurations vary between tumours and sometimes within the same tumour mass. In solid tumours epidermoid and intermediate cells usually predominate, whereas in mainly cystic tumours mucous cells tend to be more conspicuous.

Mucous cells are cuboidal, columnar or more goblet-like and form solid masses or line cysts. The mucous cells may form a single layer or be multilayered, particularly where they cover papillary projections into the cyst lumen. The mucin can be visualized with an appropriate stain such as mucicarmine or periodic acid-Schiff stain and this is sometimes useful when mucous cells are sparse. Cysts can distend and rupture into the surrounding tissue where the mucus evokes an inflammatory reaction or occasionally a more granulomatous reaction with cholesterol clefts and associated giant cells.

Epidermoid (squamous) cells usually have identifiable intercellular bridges but keratinization is very rare. They may be arranged as solid masses or form part of the cyst lining.

Intermediate cells are small with dark-staining nuclei and they often form the stratified lining of cysts below a layer of mucous cells.

Hydropic degeneration in the epidermoid cells can produce areas of clear cells, and occasionally these are the predominant feature. Rarely, mucoepidermoid carcinomas show focal or complete oncocytic metaplasia.

All mucoepidermoid carcinomas should be regarded as malignant and able to metastasize, regardless of their macroscopical or microscopical appearances. Tumours can be classified into low- and high-grade categories which provide some indication of the probable prognosis with respect to local recurrence and metastatic potential. It should however, be emphasized that these gradings form part of a spectrum of histological appearances, and although the features described provide a good guide to local behaviour, they are individually not absolute.

The *well-differentiated type* or *low-grade tumour* is usually circumscribed but non-encapsulated and predominantly cystic. More than 50% of the tumour consists of mucus-producing cells and well-differentiated epidermoid cells. Typically the tumours are less than 4 cm in diameter. Microscopy shows well-differentiated mucous cells, epidermoid cells and intermediate cells with absent or occasional mitoses and minimal nuclear pleomorphism. The margin is infiltrative, but on a broad pushing margin rather than the infiltrative permeation seen in the high grade tumours.

The *poorly differentiated type* or *high-grade tumour* is usually but not invariably more than 4 cm in diameter. These tumours have a macroscopically ill-defined margin, tend to be solid and may show focal areas of haemorrhage or necrosis. Cystic areas are usually smaller than in low-grade tumours. Microscopy shows cytological features of malignancy with a high mitotic frequency, nuclear pleomorphism and infiltrative margins. The bulk of the tumour usually consists of undifferentiated intermediate cells or poorly differentiated epidermoid cells in which it is often difficult to see the intercellular bridges. Mucous cells are rare – less than 10% – and not readily identified without special stains.

The overall 5-year survival rate is about 70%, but this can include an over 90% 5-year survival rate for low-grade tumours and a dismal prognosis for high-grade tumours. The quality of primary surgical excision is an important factor in local recurrence and prognosis.

2.3 Adenoid Cystic Carcinoma (Figs. 49–54)

An infiltrative malignant tumour having various histological features with three growth patterns: glandular (cribriform), tubular or solid. The tumour cells are of two types: duct-lining cells and cells of myoepithelial type. Perineural or perivascular spread without stromal reaction is very characteristic. All structural types of adenoid cystic carcinoma can be associated in the same tumour.

The *glandular (cribriform) type* consists of epithelial cell nests permeated by numerous cylindrical spaces (so-called Swiss-cheese spaces and sieve-like configurations). Most of these are pseudocysts (pseudolumens) containing proteoglycans and basal membrane-like material. The cells surrounding the pseudocysts resemble modified myoepithelial cells of a flat, spindle-like shape with scanty cytoplasm. The true cysts with usually inconspicuous lumens contain secretory material and are surrounded by duct-like cuboidal cells with broader, eosinophilic cytoplasm.

The *tubular type* consists of epithelial ductular structures or strands surrounded by hyaline desmoplastic stroma. Tubular lumens are lined by luminal duct-type cells, which are in turn surrounded by one or more peripheral layers of modified myoepithelial cells.

The *solid type* is characterized by solid epithelial strands. Neoplastic cell nests contain few gland-like spaces and often central necrosis. The tumor cells are small and basophilic with hyperchromatic dense nuclei. Mitoses are few. Between the cell nests there are narrow areas of stromal tissue.

All adenoid cystic carcinomas, regardless of their histological types, are biologically aggressive and can give rise to metastases many years after excision of the primary tumour. Perineural spread, perivascular spread, mitotic activity and pleomorphism appear to have no exact correlation to prognosis. Statistically, tumours of the glandular or tubular type have a better prognosis with regard to length of survival of the patient, whereas the solid type seems to have the worst prognosis, characterized by numerous early recurrences, early metastases and frequent fatal evolution. Local extension into bone appears to indicate a poor prognosis. Other important prognostic factors are the adequacy of the margin of excision and the size of the tumour. Fifty per cent of patients are alive and well at 10 years with tumours of 2 cm and under. In differential diagnosis the solid type must be distinguished from basal cell adenocarcinoma (see Sect. 2.6).

2.4 Polymorphous Low Grade Adenocarcinoma (Terminal Duct Carcinoma) (Figs. 55–60)

A malignant epithelial tumour characterized by cytological uniformity, morphological diversity and a low metastatic potential.

Macroscopically the tumour may appear to be circumscribed but microscopy shows invasion of the surrounding tissues and no evidence of encapsulation.

The cells are often pale, giving the impression under microscopy at low power that the section has been understained. They are small to medium sized and the oval nuclei are pale and vesicular with only occasional nucleoli. Mitoses are uncommon.

The striking feature of these neoplasms is the variety of morphological configurations between tumours and within an individual tumour. The main microscopical patterns are: (1) lobular, sometimes with a peripheral palisade of columnar cells, (2) papillary or papillary-cystic, (3) cribriform areas, sometimes closely resembling those in adenoid cystic carcinoma, and (4) trabeculae or small, duct-like structures, occasionally with intratubular calcification. Sometimes the cells form concentric whorls or targetoid arrangements around nerves and blood vessels. Neurotropism may be a conspicuous feature and is easily misinterpreted as indicative of adenoid cystic carcinoma. The stroma may show areas of mucinosis, hyalinization with collagen or elastic tissue and areas of haemorrhage.

The tumour appears to arise only in the minor salivary glands, particularly the palate. Despite the microscopical evidence of invasion and the disturbing neurotropism, the prognosis is good. There is local recurrence in about 20% of cases but regional and distant metastases are uncommon.

The main differential diagnosis is from papillary cystadenocarcinoma, adenoid cystic carcinoma and carcinoma in pleomorphic adenoma.

2.5 Epithelial-Myoepithelial Carcinoma (Figs. 61–63)

A tumour composed of variable proportions of two cell types which typically form duct-like structures. There is an inner layer of duct lining cells and an outer layer of clear cells.

The tumour is usually multinodular. It may be encapsulated, but the capsule is frequently incomplete and tumour nodules often extend through it.

The inner layer of the duct-like structures consists of small, dark-staining, cuboidal cells. The outer clear cells stain strongly for glycogen and are also positive for S-100 protein and myosin. Electron microscopy also shows features consistent with a myoepithelial origin. There is considerable variation in the proportion of duct lining cells and clear cells, and occasionally the latter are the predominant feature, forming sheets or nests of clear cells rather than duct-like structures. Mitoses are rare and the tumour is cytologically bland; indeed, it has previously been classified as a type of adenoma. However, perineural and vascular invasion may be present and recurrence and metastasis are not uncommon.

This is essentially a tumour confined to the major glands, particularly to the parotid (80%), with a peak incidence in later life (7th and 8th decades).

The differential diagnosis from other clear cell tumours of salivary glands is discussed in the Introduction.

2.6 Basal Cell Adenocarcinoma (Figs. 64–68)

An epithelial neoplasm that has cytological characteristics of basal cell adenoma but morphological growth pattern indicative of malignancy.

The cytological features of individual cells and the general morphological features of basal cell adenocarcinoma are markedly similar to those of basal cell adenoma; in fact, aside from those few cases with a mitotic index so high that a malignant diagnosis can be considered on this feature alone, it may be impossible to differentiate basal cell adenoma from basal cell adenocarcinoma cytologically. The growth character of the tumour in relation to the surrounding tissues is the key feature used to distinguish adenoma from carcinoma in basal cell salivary gland neoplasms.

These tumours have a uniform, monomorphic appearance like that of basal cell carcinomas or eccrine cylindromas of the skin. Two forms of epithelial cell are observed and are usually intermingled with one another. One is a small, round cell with scant cytoplasm and a dark basophilic nucleus. The other is a larger, polygonal to elongated cell with eosinophilic or amphophilic cytoplasm and a larger, pale basophilic nucleus. In both types the cell-to-cell boundaries are indistinct. Frequently, palisading of the nuclei occurs along the epithelial-stromal interface. Pale cells sometimes appear to form swirls or eddies within the islands of tumour and may have a squamoid appearance and occasionally keratinize. Small tubules or lumens can be seen in many of the epithelial islands and may be prominent in focal areas. Eosinophilic and periodic acid-Schiff-positive, hyaline material may be seen as coalescing, intercellular droplets and membranes surrounding individual tumour islands. This latter feature may produce a marked resemblance to dermal cylindromas, especially in those tumours categorized as membranous type basal cell adenocarcinomas, but histological patterns can resemble any of the subtypes of basal cell adenoma (see Sect. 1.3).

In accordance with the histological patterns described for basal cell adenomas, basal cell adenocarcinomas can be divided into four subtypes: solid, trabecular, tubular, and membranous.

The *solid type* is characterized by contiguous tumour cells arranged in islands and masses within the fibrous connective tissue stroma. In some lesions these basaloid epithelial cells form numerous small tumour islands that tend to be round to oval shaped. In other tumours of the solid type the epithelium forms large irregular masses.

The *membranous type* is distinguished by thick eosinophilic, periodic acid-Schiff-positive hyaline lamina that surround and separate tumour nests and may create a jigsaw puzzle appearance in portions of the tumour.

Anastomosing cords and bands of basaloid epithelial cells characterize the *trabecular type* of basal cell adenocarcinoma. These interconnecting cords may be likened to the Chinese character-like configurations formed by bone trabeculae in fibrous dysplasia of bone.

Conspicuous small lumina or pseudolumina characterize the *tubular type* of basal cell adenocarcinoma. These lumina are not surrounded by intralobular or interlobular type ductal cells but by basal cells that blend indistinctly with adjacent basal cells that do not bound lumina. The lumina appear to be more like tiny cystic spaces than true duct lumina.

Salivary gland mucin is absent or present in insignificant amounts within all of these types of basal cell adenocarcinoma. The periodic acid-Schiff stain nicely highlights the basal lamina material in and around the tumour cell nests.

The distinctive diagnostic feature that separates these adenocarcinomas from typical benign basal cell adenomas is invasive growth. Nests and strands of tumour cells insinuate into the salivary gland lobules between the acini and/or into the adjacent structures such as skeletal muscle, fat and dermis. About a third of the tumours display perineural invasion, and nearly a quarter exhibit intravascular invasion.

Basal cell adenocarcinomas are low grade adenocarcinomas with a relatively good prognosis. Recurrence is relatively frequent, but metastasis is less common, usually to regional lymph nodes. Only one death has been documented in the literature at this time.

This category of salivary gland tumour has only recently been clearly defined, and this entity was not included in the first edition of the classification. Although cumulative experience is small, one series has estimated its frequency at about 4% of all primary parotid gland carcinomas. Basal cell adenocarcinoma has no sex predilection. It has not been described in children and most patients are over 50 years old. Basal cell adenocarcinoma occurs predominantly in the parotid gland, less frequently in the submandibular gland, and is distinctly rare in minor salivary glands.

2.7 Sebaceous Carcinoma (Figs. 69, 70)

A rare variety of carcinoma composed of sebaceous cells of varying degrees of maturity.

There are two types of carcinoma in this category:

Sebaceous carcinoma is almost exclusively found in the parotid gland. It consists of nests and sheets of sebaceous cells with various degrees of cellular atypia and some mitoses.

Sebaceous lymphadenocarcinoma is a very rare distinctive variety of sebaceous carcinoma composed of areas of sebaceous lymphadenoma with an adjacent malignant carcinomatous component. It is the malignant counterpart of sebaceous lymphadenoma, with the same problems in regard to histogenesis (see Sect. 1.7).

Sebaceous carcinomas appear to be low grade malignant tumours with the ability to recur locally. They may also develop lymph node and, exceptionally, distant metastases.

2.8 Papillary Cystadenocarcinoma (Figs. 71, 72)

A malignant tumour characterized by cysts and papillary endocystic projections.

Papillary cystadenocarcinoma is composed of one or several cystic spaces filled with papillae. These papillae have narrow, fibrous, sometimes hyalinized cores, covered with cuboidal or low columnar cells. Mucous secreting cells can be present. Malignancy is confirmed by nuclear pleomorphism, mitoses and infiltrative growth.

Papillary cystadenocarcinoma is a low grade carcinoma.

Papillary cystadenocarcinoma must be distinguished from benign papillary cystadenoma (see Sect. 1.9.1) and other carcinomas which show papillary structures. Immunohistochemistry can be useful to eliminate a diagnosis of metastasis of papillary thyroid carcinoma.

2.9 Mucinous Adenocarcinoma (Figs. 73, 74)

A rare tumour characterized by abundant mucus production.
   Cuboidal or columnar cells line mucus-filled lumens or cysts. The mucus should occupy over 50% of the tumour. Epidermoid or intermediate cells are not present.

2.10 Oncocytic Carcinoma (Figs. 75–77)

A very rare tumour composed of malignant oncocytic cells.
   Two groups of criteria are necessary to establish a diagnosis of oncocytic carcinoma. First, the tumour cells must be identified as oncocytes (see Sect. 1.5). Second, the diagnosis of malignancy should be based not only on cellular and nuclear pleomorphism (occasionally seen in benign oncocytoma) but also on local infiltration, perineural or vascular infiltration or metastasis.
   Oncocytic carcinoma can recur locally and may develop lymph node or distant metastases. Prognosis seems to be related to tumour size.

2.11 Salivary Duct Carcinoma (Figs. 78, 79)

An epithelial tumour of high malignancy with formation of relatively large cell aggregates resembling distended salivary ducts. The neoplastic epithelium presents a combination of cribriform, looping ('Roman bridging') and solid growth patterns, often with central necrosis both in the primary lesions and the lymph node metastases.
   This extremely rare carcinoma resembles comedocarcinoma of the breast. Neoplastic cells display an eosinophilic cytoplasm, often with an apocrine appearance. Staining with mucicarmine and alcian blue usually gives negative results. Nuclear pleomorphism and frequent mitoses are present. The stroma can be fibrous and desmoplastic.
   The generally poor prognosis of this tumour justifies diagnostic separation from other carcinomas of the salivary glands. At surgery, the tumour is usually found to infiltrate adjacent tissues and involve cervical lymph nodes. The majority of patients die within 3 years. The tumour occurs almost exclusively in the parotid.

Salivary duct carcinoma must be differentiated from high grade mucoepidermoid carcinoma, which contains mucous secreting cells, from oncocytic carcinoma, and particularly from polymorphous low grade adenocarcinoma, which has a much better prognosis.

2.12 Adenocarcinoma

A carcinoma with glandular, ductal or secretory differentiation that does not fit into the other categories of carcinoma.

2.13 Malignant Myoepithelioma (Myoepithelial Carcinoma)
(Figs. 80–83)

A rare malignant epithelial tumour composed of atypical myoepithelial cells (see Sect. 1.2) with increased mitotic activity and aggressive growth.

The cytological features of individual cells and the general morphological features are very similar to benign myoepithelioma and the myoepithelial cells of pleomorphic adenoma. The tumour cells may be spindle-shaped or more rounded, sometimes with eosinophilic cytoplasm and eccentric nuclei, so-called hyaline or plasmacytoid cells. The cell types are often intermixed, but usually one or the other cell type predominates. The tumours may be quite cellular and easily confused with sarcoma. The stroma in other areas of the tumours may be more conspicuous and myxoid.

These tumours are distinguished from benign myoepithelial neoplasms by their infiltrative, destructive growth. They may also demonstrate mitotic activity and cytological pleomorphism.

Although reactions may be variable, immunohistochemistry can help to identify the myoepithelial nature of these tumours. Some tumour cells should be immunoreactive for cytokeratin, S-100 protein, smooth muscle actin, and, occasionally, glial fibrillary acidic protein (GFAP).

Myoepithelial carcinomas are very uncommon neoplasms that have only rarely been reported in the literature. Most tumours have occurred in the parotid gland of adults over 50 years old. While this tumour is locally destructive, metastasis is infrequent.

2.14 Carcinoma in Pleomorphic Adenoma
(Malignant Mixed Tumour) (Figs. 84–89)

Tumours showing definitive evidence of malignancy, such as cyto-
logical and histological characteristics of anaplasia, abnormal mi-
toses, progressive course and infiltrative growth, and in which evi-
dence of pleomorphic adenoma can still be found.

The development of a secondary carcinoma in a pre-existing pleomorphic adenoma can be observed in 3%–4% of all pleomorphic
adenomas. The incidence of malignancy shows a correlation between
the length of history of pleomorphic adenoma and the development
of a carcinoma. The risk of developing malignancy is only about 1.5%
up to 5 years, but increases to 9.5% after more than 15 years.

Concerning infiltrative growth and pathohistological differentiation, three subtypes can be distinguished: non-invasive carcinoma in
pleomorphic adenoma, invasive carcinoma in pleomorphic adenoma
and carcinosarcoma (true malignant mixed tumour).

The term *"non-invasive carcinoma"* refers to circumscribed malignant areas in a pleomorphic adenoma without infiltration of the
surrounding tissue. This term is preferred to "intracapsular carcinoma" or "carcinoma in situ". Patients with non-invasive carcinoma
have an excellent prognosis if the tumour is completely removed
surgically.

In *invasive carcinomas* the extent of invasion as measured in mil-
limeters is a valuable guide to prognosis and biological behaviour:
carcinomas invading less than 8 mm carry a 5-year survival of 100%,
carcinomas invading more than 8 mm a 5-year survival of less than
50%. Findings suggestive of malignant changes in pleomorphic
adenoma are micronecrosis, haemorrhage, calcification and/or excessive hyalinization. Sites of metastases are lymph nodes, lung and
bone. The main types of carcinomas arising in pleomorphic adenomas are undifferentiated carcinoma, ductal carcinoma or polymorphous low grade adenocarcinoma. The carcinomas of high grade
malignancy carry a worse prognosis with regard to the survival time.

Carcinosarcomas are very rare and are made up of carcinomatous and sarcomatous features. The sarcomatous component shows
mostly a chondrosarcomatous pattern. This true biphasic tumour is
highly lethal, with a 5-year survival of 0%. Metastases from carcinosarcoma usually contain both tissue components.

The most unusual and rarest variant is the *metastasizing pleomor-*
phic adenoma, defined as a histologically benign tumour that inex-

plicably manifests distant mestastases. The primary salivary gland tumour and its metastases are composed of "benign" mixed tumour structures.

2.15 Squamous Cell Carcinoma (Fig. 90)

A malignant epithelial tumour with cells forming keratin or having intercellular bridges. Mucus secretion is not present.

Distinguishing between primary squamous cell carcinoma of the salivary gland and metastases of primary squamous cell carcinoma of the skin is difficult because the histological appearance in each case is similar (see Sect. 5). The diagnosis may rest on clinical data.

2.16 Small Cell Carcinoma (Figs. 91, 92)

A malignant tumour similar in histology, behaviour and histochemistry to the small cell carcinoma of the lung.

By electron microscopy two types of small cell carcinoma can be distinguished: a neuroendocrine variety with small, dense-core endocrine granules and strong immunoreactivity for neuron-specific enolase or chromogranin, and a ductal variety without endocrine organelles. The diagnosis of small cell carcinoma of the salivary gland should be made only after excluding the possibility of a primary tumour arising in the lung (see Sect. 5).

2.17 Undifferentaited Carcinoma (Figs. 93, 94)

A malignant tumour of epithelial structure that is too poorly differentiated, i. e. is devoid of any phenotypic expression by light microscopy, to be placed in any of the other groups of carcinoma.

The tumour cells may be predominantly spheroidal (large cells) or spindle-shaped. Cell size and ultrastructural features have little bearing on prognosis. The single most important clinicopathological factor relating to outcome is size of the primary tumour. Carcinomas larger than 4 cm carry the poorest prognosis.

A special subtype is the *undifferentiated carcinoma with lymphoid stroma.* This tumour is characterized by syncytial clumps of large cells with vesicular nuclei and prominent nucleoli, admixed with abundant small lymphocytes and plasma cells. This tumor has a relatively high incidence in Inuits and Chinese and was described as 'malignant lymphoepithelial lesion of the salivary gland'. It has been suggested that Epstein-Barr virus may have an role in its development. The tumour is histologically indistinguishable from the lymphoepithelial undifferentiated carcinoma of the nasopharynx. It is therefore essential to examine the upper respiratory tract and to obtain biopsy specimens from the nasopharynx before accepting the diagnosis of a primary undifferentiated carcinoma of the salivary glands.

2.18 Other Carcinomas (Figs. 95–97)

Like carcinoma in pleomorphic adenoma (see Sect. 2.14), the development of *carcinoma in a Warthin tumour* is observed very rarely. Reported cases have been mostly squamous cell carcinoma, mucoepidermoid carcinoma or acinic cell carcinoma. Metastatic carcinoma in a Warthin tumour must be excluded.

Embryonal carcinoma, a neoplastic proliferation of the cell system of one organ anlage with variable differentiation, is very rare. The tumour includes ductular epithelial structures of varying architecture, acinar cell groups with amylase granules and more highly differentiated parts similar to a pleomorphic adenoma.

Whether a primary *adenosquamous carcinoma* of minor salivary glands exists is controversial. Adenocarcinomatous and squamous carcinomatous components should be present in a single tumour with intercellular bridges or keratin demonstrable in the squamous component. Adenocarcinomas with small foci of squamous differentiation should be classified as adenocarcinomas.

3 Non-epithelial Tumours (Figs. 98–100)

Non-epithelial tumours are classified according to the WHO *Histological Classification of Soft Tissue Tumours.*[1]

---

[1] Enzinger FM, Lattes R, Torloni H (1969) Histological Typing of Soft Tissue Tumours. International Histological Classification of Tumours, No. 3. WHO, Geneva

Non-epithelial tumours make up 5% of all tumours of the salivary glands.

Men seem to be predisposed to lipomas (85%), neural tumours (60%) and sarcomas (65%). About 90% of non-epithelial tumours are benign.

The most common type of benign mesenchymal tumour is angioma (45%), especially haemangioma or lymphangioma, rarely haemangiopericytoma. Angiomas represent about 50% of salivary gland tumours in children but less than 5% in adults.

Lipomas represent about 20% of all benign mesenchymal tumours of the salivary glands, as do neural tumours (neurinoma, neurofibroma, neurofibromatosis).

The age peak for angiomas is in the 1st and 2nd decades of life, while lipomas occur in the 4th and 5th decades. Neural tumours show a relatively even distribution from the 3rd to the 6th decade.

Sarcomas most frequently appear in the form of malignant fibrous histiocytoma, malignant schwannoma or rhabdomyosarcoma.

4 Malignant Lymphomas (Figs. 101–103)

The lymphoid tissue of salivary glands can be considered as part of the mucosa-associated lymphoid tissue (MALT), but also shows features of the peripheral lymphoid tissue similar to the Waldeyer ring. The lymphoid tissue consists of intra-epithelial lymphocytes, lymphocytes and plasma cells diffusely distributed in the glandular parenchyma and intra- or periglandular lymph nodes, especially of the parotid or submandibular gland.

Malignant lymphomas can involve the salivary glands as the only manifestation of the disease or as a part of systemic spread. The standard minimum criteria for acceptance of a salivary gland lymphoma as primary are: no palpable superficial lympadenopathy at presentation, no enlargement of mediastinal lymph nodes in chest X-rays, normal white cell count and no manifestation in other lymph nodes, gut, liver or spleen.

Malignant lymphomas of the salivary glands are usually associated with chronic immunosialadenitis (benign lymphoepithelial lesion, Sjögren syndrome; see Sect. 7.4). The risk of development of a malignant lymphoma in patients with Sjögren syndrome is 40 times higher than in the normal population.

The large majority of salivary gland lymphomas are of the non-Hodgkin type (85%) and should be classified using the same terminology as is applied to lymphoid tissues. Two-thirds are well differentiated (immunocytomas, centrocytic-centroblastic lymphomas, lymphoplasmacytic, plasmacytic and follicular centre cleaved cell types). The poorly differentiated lymphomas are dominated by the immunoblastic lymphoma. Hodgkin lymphoma constitutes only 15% of malignant lymphomas of the salivary glands. The lymphocyte-predominant and nodular-sclerosing forms are more common than the lymphocyte-depleted forms, which have a worse prognosis.

About 5% of all extranodal lymphomas affect the salivary glands. About 40% of malignant lymphomas of the head and neck arise in the salivary glands.

5 Secondary Tumours (Figs. 104, 105)

The distinction between malignant primary tumours of the salivary glands and metastases to the salivary glands is of practical importance for therapy and prognosis. This distinction is particularly difficult with the following types: small cell carcinoma, undifferentiated carcinoma of the nasopharyngeal type with lymphoid stroma, mammary, lobular or ductal carcinomas, clear cell carcinomas, and squamous cell carcinomas.

About 40% of metastatic tumours are localized in the glandular parenchyma and 60% in the lymph nodes of the salivary glands. The architecture of the lymphatic vessels and the number of intraglandular lymph nodes play an important role in the propagation of tumour cells in the parotid gland. Between 20 and 30 lymph nodes are found in the parotid region, but no intraglandular lymph nodes are in the submandibular gland. Most metastases to the salivary glands develop from primary squamous cell carcinomas of the skin (head and neck) or from melanomas of this region. Rarely, metastases occur from nasopharyngeal carcinomas, and, very rarely, metastases from thyroid carcinomas. About 75% of these metastases are localized in the parotid gland.

Haematogenous metastases in the salivary glands (usually to the parotid or submandibular glands) are relatively rare. They are mainly from three sites: lung, kidney and breast. Small cell carcinomas of the salivary gland are more likely to be metastatic than primary. In some cases, the application of immunocytochemical techniques may be of considerable help: the presence of thyroglobulin indicates a thyroid neoplasm, while hormone receptors may act as useful markers for mammary carcinomas.

6 Unclassified Tumours

Benign or malignant tumours that cannot be placed in any of the categories described above.

7 Tumour-like Lesions

Certain lesions may present as swellings or induration of the salivary glands thought on clinical grounds to be tumours.

7.1 Sialadenosis (Fig. 106)

Sialadenosis is a non-inflammatory salivary disease due to metabolic and secretory disorders of the gland parenchyma accompanied by recurrent painless bilateral swelling, usually of the parotid glands. The lesion has been related to endocrine disorders (diabetes mellitus, ovarian and thyroid insufficiencies), malnutrition, chronic alcoholism, liver cirrhosis and dysfunction of the autonomic nervous system. Sialadenosis is a disorder of the salivary gland innervation with peripheral autonomic neuropathy.

Histologically there is enlargement of the serous acinar cells and slight compression of the duct system by the swollen acini. The nuclei of the acinar cells are displaced toward to the basal part of the cell. On the basis of the content of mature periodic acid-Schiff-positive enzyme granules, three types of sialadenosis can be distinguished: granular (dense filling of the cytoplasm with granules); honeycomb with vacuolated cytoplasm; and mixed. Unlike in the benign lymphoepithelial lesion, there are no inflammatory cells.

Electron microscopy shows atrophic changes of the myoepithelial cells and degeneration of the autonomic nervous system (loss of neurosecretory granules, axolysis, etc.).

7.2 Oncocytosis (Figs. 107–109)

Diffuse oncocytosis of the parotid gland is a very rare non-neoplastic lesion due to complete oncocytic metaplasia of the gland lobules affecting both the ductal and acinar epithelium. This is an intracellular metabolic disorder with mitochondriopathy. Diffuse oncocytosis is almost always unilateral, unlike sialadenosis, and occurs in older age groups.

Multifocal oncocytic adenomatous hyperplasia is a non-encapsulated, partly micronodular and partly macronodular hyperplasia of oncocytic buds from the ductal epithelium. Remnants of the original salivary tissue with acini and fatty tissue are usually present between the oncocytic foci. It is assumed that oncocytoma can arise by confluent growth and later formation of a capsule (see Sect. 1.5).

7.3 Necrotizing Sialometaplasia (Salivary Gland Infarction) (Figs. 110–113)

This is an ischaemic lesion mostly localized in the palate. The term 'salivary gland infarction' is based upon the fact that the lesion resembles infarcts in other organs, such as the prostate gland.

Histologically the lesion shows a lobular arrangement with squamous cell metaplasia of the duct system in the centre. Necrotic acini and inflammatory resorptive cell infiltrates are found peripherally. These are usually surrounded by intact glandular tissue. Vascular changes have been described around the salivary gland infarct, including stenosis, thrombosis, or obliteration of blood vessels, particularly after operations.

The lesion must be distinguished from squamous cell carcinoma. Goblet cells may occur within the squamous cell metaplasia, a finding that can lead to confusion with mucoepidermoid carcinoma.

7.4 Benign Lymphoepithelial Lesion (Figs. 114, 115)

The histopathological appearance of this lesion is made up of a triad of parenchymatous atrophy, interstitial lymphocytic infiltration, and so-called epimyoepithelial cell islands. The development of the epimyoepithelial cell islands shows different phases, initially with lumen remnants, later with an increase of lymphocytic infiltration and finally hyaline transformation.

The disease affects older women almost exclusively and is characterized by a recurrent painful swelling mostly of the parotid glands. It is regarded as an autoimmune disease of the salivary glands. The alteration can be observed as a local disorder of the salivary gland ('myoepithelial sialadenitis') or a manifestation of Sjögren syndrome. In the latter case the patients often have rheumatoid arthritis (or other connective tissue disorders), keratoconjunctivitis sicca and xerostomia. The minor salivary glands, particularly those of the lip, are inflamed in addition to the major glands. Histological examination shows duct ectasia, lymphocytic infiltrate, and marked sclerosis of glands with atrophy of acini and destruction of the lobules. Epimyoepithelial islands are rarely found in the minor salivary glands.

The risk of development of a malignant lymphoma, especially non-Hodgkin lymphoma, increases to 40:1 in patients with Sjögren syndrome, particularly where there is a long history of a pre-existing benign lymphoepithelial lesion (see Sect. 4).

7.5 Salivary Gland Cysts (Figs. 116–120)

Non-neoplastic cysts form about 6% of all lesions of the salivary glands and cause localized swelling which may resemble neoplasms.

More than 75% are found to be in the minor salivary glands as mucoceles. Most common are *extravasated cysts*, mainly in the lower lip. The extravasation of mucus into the interstitium results in a mucus-filled pseudocyst with a connective tissue capsule and resorptive cell infiltration including macrophages and foreign body giant cells. By contrast, the *retention cyst* is less common and has an epithelial lining, a retained mucous mass which is finely flocculated and may also contain spheroliths or microliths.

Salivary duct cysts occur mainly in the parotid gland and constitute about 10% of all cysts of the salivary glands. Similar to the retention cyst, the salivary duct cysts are lined by duct epithelium and contain mucus.

Lymphoepithelial cysts develop mainly in the parotid gland, but also in the floor of the mouth. The cysts are bordered by a flattened multilayered epithelium that is always surrounded by a lymphoid stroma with lymph follicles. Sometimes the cysts are lined by squamous epithelium with keratinization on the surface. The cysts contain a serous fluid with inclusions of desquamated epithelium, lymphocytes and foam cells. The synonymous term 'branchiogenic parotid cyst' should be avoided because the histogenetic development from the branchial region is not definitely established.

Dysgenetic polycystic disease of the parotid gland is a very rare disorder resembling cystic anomalies of other organs, such as the kidney, liver, pancreas or lung. Histologically it is characterized by various duct-type cysts lined by epithelium. The duct lumen contains secretion with inclusion of spheroliths or microliths. Remnants of gland tissue with acini can be observed between the cysts, but inflammatory changes are absent.

7.6 Chronic Sclerosing Sialadenitis of Submandibular Gland (Küttner Tumour) (Fig. 121)

This is an inflammatory process producing a firm, swollen submandibular gland that often cannot be distinguished from a true tumour. In progressive stages the histological features are periductal sclerosis and dense lymphocytic infiltration, reduction of the secretory gland parenchyma, development of secondary lymph follicles with reactive germinal centers, clumps of secretion in the ducts, ductular proliferation and destruction of the lobular architecture (so-called salivary gland cirrhosis). Pathogenetic factors include a disorder of secretion, obstruction of the duct system by sialoliths, lymphocytic inflammation and immune reactions of the duct system.

7.7 Cystic Lymphoid Hyperplasia in AIDS (Figs. 122–124)

Involvement of the salivary gland lymph nodes, especially those of the parotid gland, accounts for most AIDS-related cases of salivary gland enlargement. This may be associated with a Sjögren syndrome-like illness.

The pathological features consist of lymphoid tissue changes analogous to those described in persistent generalized lymphadenopathy (hypervascular reactive lymphoid hyperplasia) and in association with gross epithelial cysts within lymph nodes. The confluent cystic cavities are filled with a mucous and gelatinous substance. The

cystic spaces are lined by tonsil-like invaginating squamous epithelium of variable thickness. The metaplastic squamous epithelium is
derived from salivary duct inclusions within lymph nodes. The increased epithelial metaplastic cystic component might represent an
exuberant reaction to HIV or another virus infection.

TNM Classification
of Salivary Gland Tumours[1]

Rules for Classification

The classification applies only to carcinoma of the major salivary glands (ICD-0 C07, C08): parotid (C07), submandibular (C08.0) and sublingual (C08.1) glands. Tumours arising in minor salivary glands (mucus-secreting glands in the lining membrane of the upper aero-digestive tract) are not included in this classification. There should be histological confirmation of the disease.

The following are the procedures for assessment of the T, N and M categories:

T categories: Physical examination and imaging
N categories: Physical examination and imaging
M categories: Physical examination and imaging

Regional Lymph Nodes

The regional lymph nodes are the cervical nodes.

[1] Hermanek P, Sobin LH (1987) TNM Classification of Malignant Tumours, 4th edn. International Union Against Cancer. Springer, Berlin Heidelberg New York

TNM Clinical Classification

T – Primary Tumour

TX   Primary tumour cannot be assessed
T0   No evidence of primary tumour
T1   Tumour 2 cm or less in greatest dimension
T2   Tumour more than 2 cm but not more than 4 cm in greatest dimension
T3   Tumour more than 4 cm but not more than 6 cm in greatest dimension
T4   Tumour more than 6 cm in greatest dimension

Note: All categories are subdivided into (a) no local extension, (b) local extension. Local extension is constituted by clinical or macroscopic evidence of invasion of skin, soft tissues, bone or nerve. Microscopic evidence alone does not constitute local extension for classification purposes.

N – Regional Lymph Nodes

NX   Regional lymph nodes cannot be assessed
N0   No regional lymph node metastasis
N1   Metastasis in a single ipsilateral lymph node, 3 cm or less in greatest dimension
N2   Metastasis in a single ipsilateral lymph node, more than 3 cm but not more than 6 cm in greatest dimension, or in multiple ipsilateral lymph nodes, none more than 6 cm in greatest dimension, or in bilateral or contralateral lymph nodes, none more than 6 cm in greatest dimension
    N2a Metastasis in a single ipsilateral lymph node, more than 3 cm but not more than 6 cm in greatest dimension
    N2b Metastasis in multiple ipsilateral lymph nodes, none more than 6 cm in greatest dimension
    N2c Metastasis in bilateral or contralateral lymph nodes, none more than 6 cm in greatest dimension
N3   Metastasis in a lymph node more than 6 cm in greatest dimension

Note: Midline nodes are considered ipsilateral nodes

M – Distant Metastasis

MX   Presence of distant metastasis cannot be assessed
M0   No distant metastasis
M1   Distant metastasis

pTNM Pathological Classification

The pT, pN and pM categories correspond to the T, N and M categories.

Stage Grouping

Stage I	T1a	N0	M0
	T2a	N0	M0
Stage II	T1b	N0	M0
	T2b	N0	M0
	T3a	N0	M0
Stage III	T3b	N0	M0
	T4a	N0	M0
	Any T (except T4b)	N1	M0
Stage IV	T4b	Any N	M0
	Any T	N2, N3	M0
	Any T	Any N	M1

Summary

Salivary Glands

T1	≤2 cm	
T2	>2 to 4 cm	Categories divided:
T3	>4 to 6 cm	(a) no extension
T4	>6 cm	(b) extension
N1	Ipsilateral single ≤3 cm	
N2	Ipsilateral single >3 to 6 cm	
	Ipsilateral multiple ≤6 cm	
	Bilateral, contralateral ≤6 cm	
N3	>6 cm	

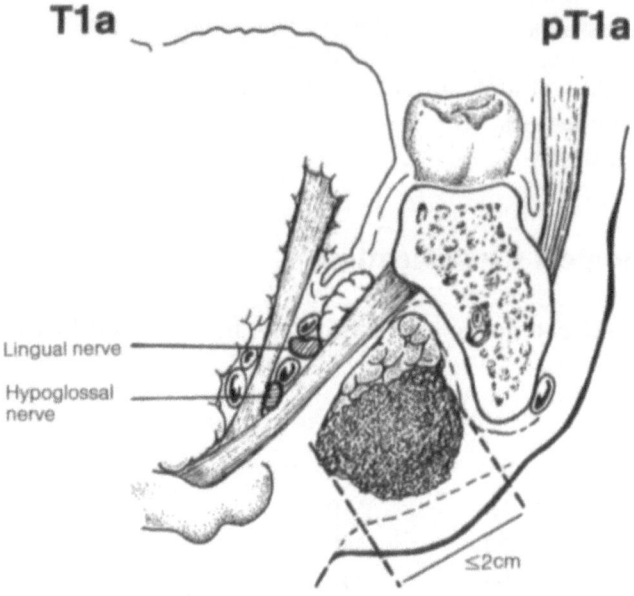

Classification determined clinically on the basis of absence of paralysis or macroscopically on the basis of no local extension (a). Frontal section through the premolar region

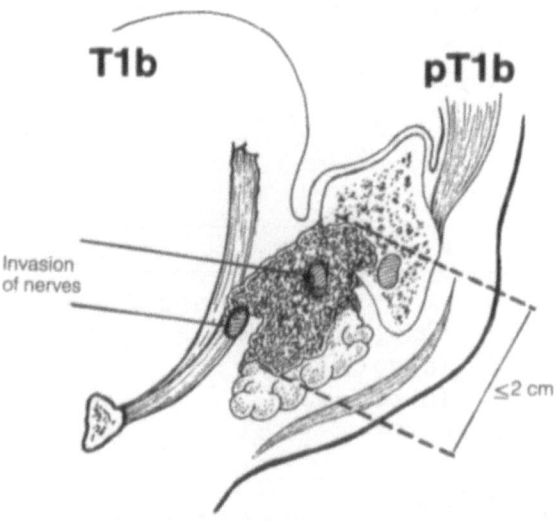

Clinical or macroscopic evidence of local extension (b). Frontal section through the retromolar region

T2   Tumour more than 2 cm but not more than 4 cm in greatest dimension

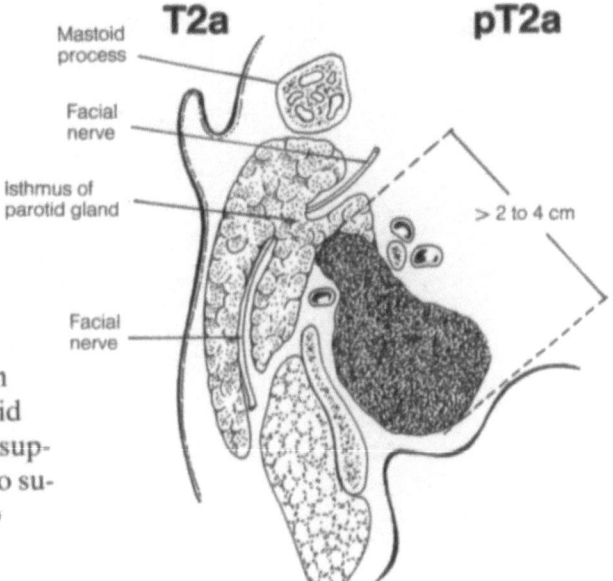

Horizontal section through the parotid gland showing its supposed division into superficial and deep lobes

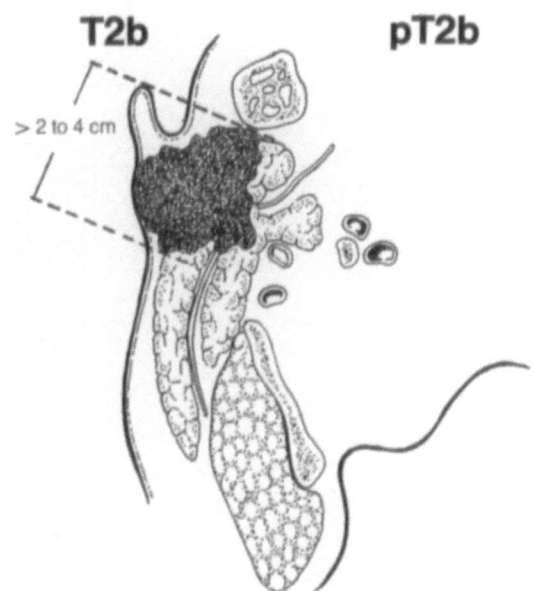

T3   Tumour more than 4 cm but not more than 6 cm in greatest
dimension

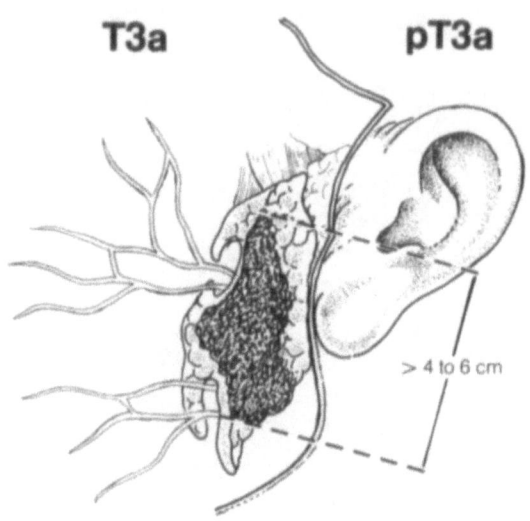

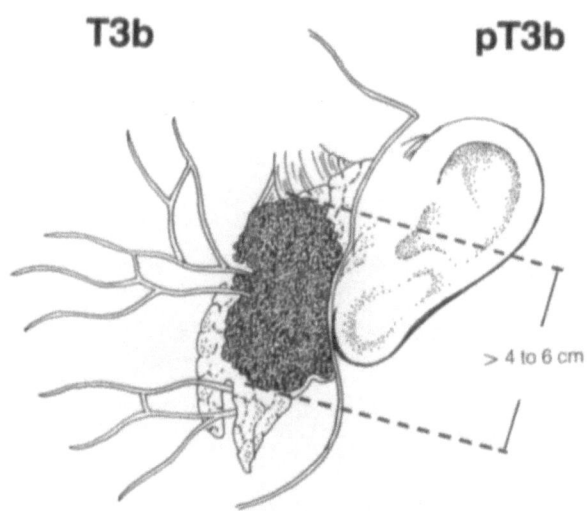

T4   Tumour more than 6 cm in greatest dimension

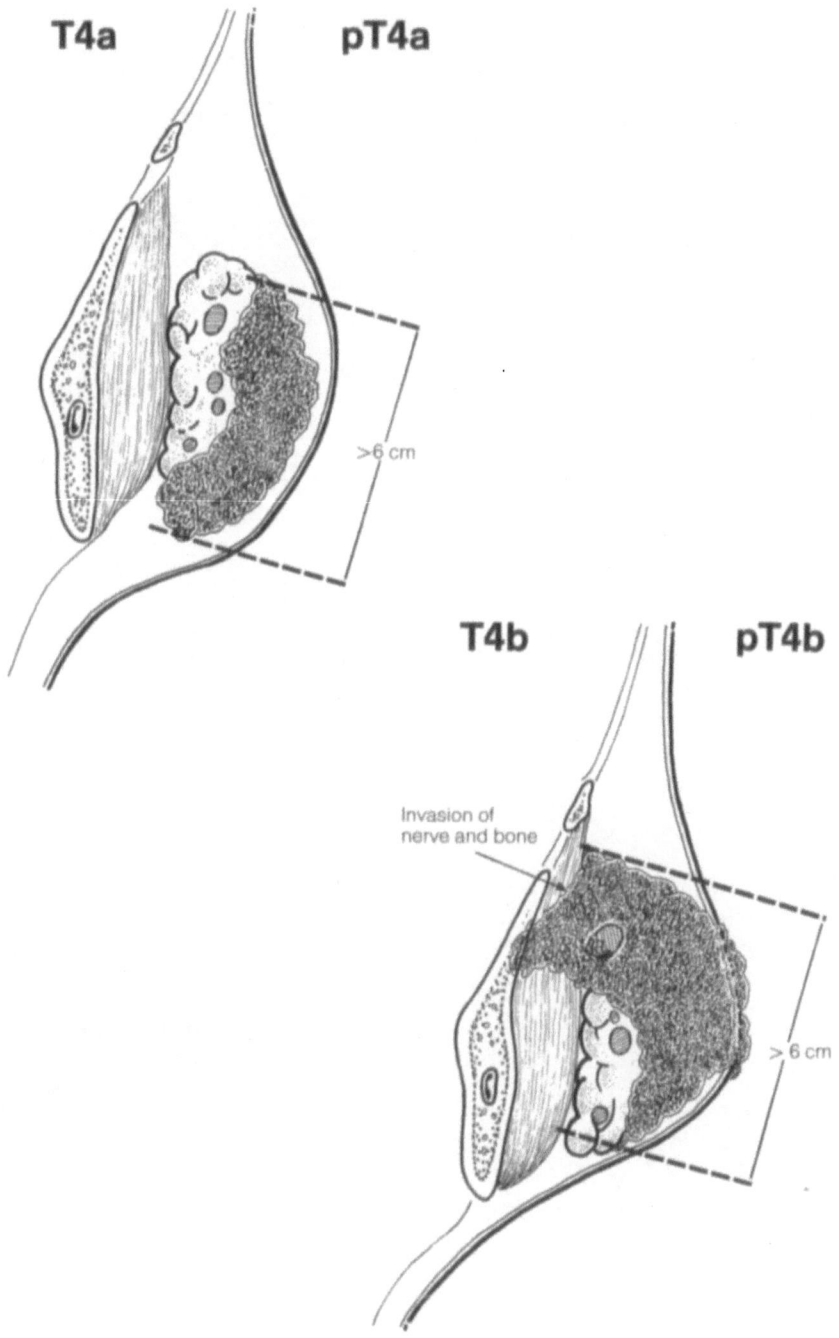

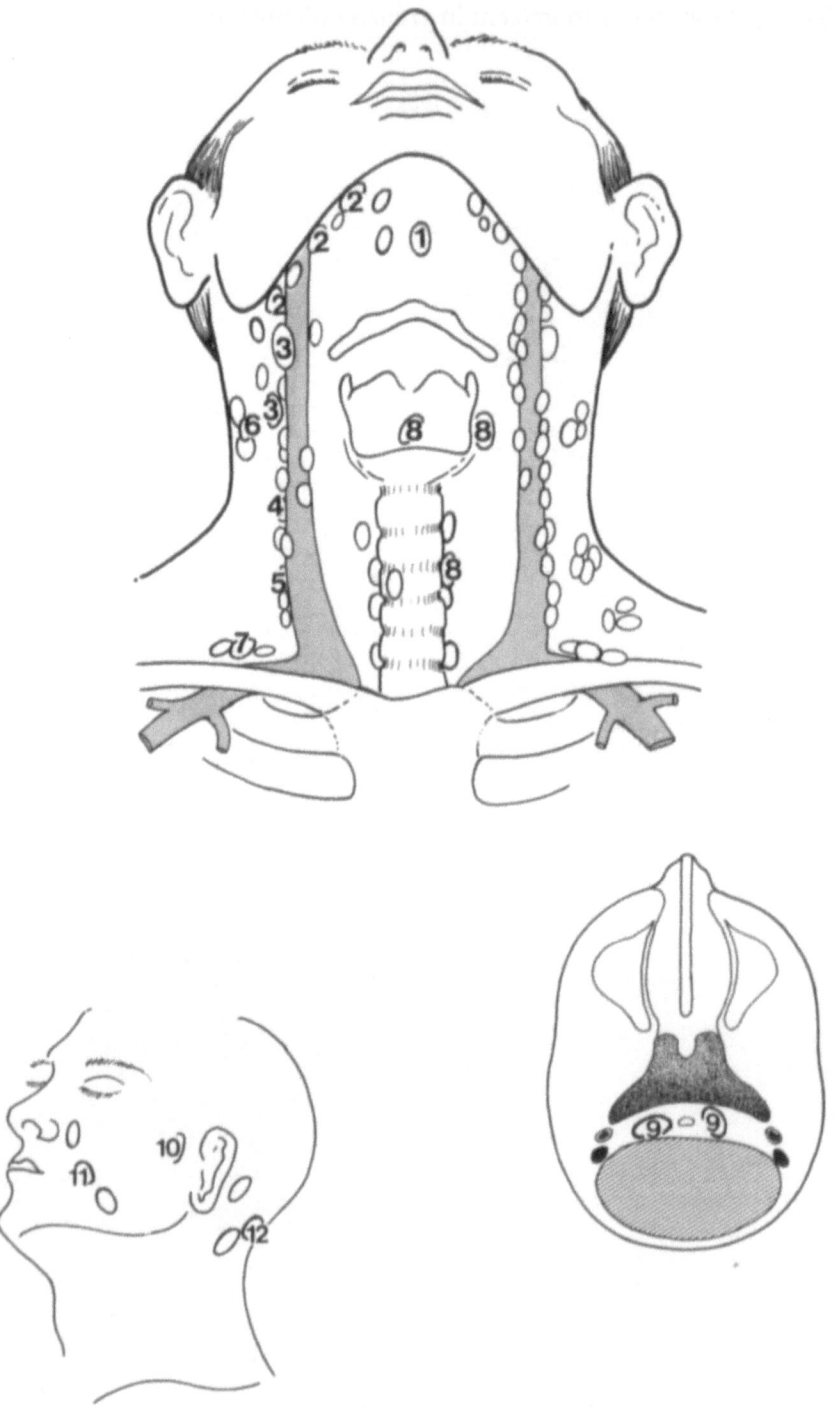

Regional Lymph Nodes

The regional lymph nodes are the cervical nodes. These include
(1) submental nodes
(2) submandibular nodes
(3) cranial jugular (deep cervical) nodes
(4) medial jugular (deep cervical) nodes
(5) caudal jugular (deep cervical) nodes
(6) dorsal cervical (superficial cervical) nodes along the accessory nerve
(7) supraclavicular nodes
(8) prelaryngeal and paratracheal nodes
(9) retropharyngeal nodes
(10) parotid nodes
(11) buccal nodes
(12) retroauricular and occipital nodes

The figures on pp 42–46 are reproduced from Spiessl B, Beahrs OH, Hermanek P, Hutter RVP, Scheibe O, Sobin LH, Wagner G (eds) (1990) TNM Atlas. Illustrated Guide to the TNM/pTNM-Classification of Malignant Tumours, 3rd edn. corrected reprint. Springer, Berlin Heidelberg New York, pp 4 and 51–54.

Subject Index

	Page	Figures
Adenocarcinoma	28	–
–, basal cell	24	64–68
–, mucinous	27	73, 74
–, polymorphous low-grade	22	55–60
Adenolymphoma, *see* Warthin Tumour		
Adenoma, basal cell	13	8–11
–, canalicular	15	20, 21
–, carcinoma in pleomorphic	29	84–89
–, metastasizing pléomorphic, *see* pleomorphic adenoma		
–, myoepithelial, *see* myoepithelioma		
–, oncocytic, *see* oncocytoma		
–, pleomorphic	11	1–5
–, sebaceous	15	22
Carcinoma, acinic cell	17	32–39
–, adenoid cystic	21	49–54
–, adenosquamous	31	–
–, embryonal	31	–
–, epithelial-myoepithelial	23	61–63
–, in pleomorphic adenoma	29	84–89
–, in Warthin tumour	31	95–97
–, mucoepidermoid	20	40–48
–, myoepithelial, *see* myoepithelioma, malignant		
–, oncocytic	27	75–77
–, other	31	95–97
–, salivary duct	27	78, 79
–, sebaceous	26	69, 70
–, small cell	30	91, 92
–, squamous cell	30	90
–, terminal duct, *see* adenocarcinoma, polymorphic low-grade		
–, undifferentiated	30	93, 94
Carcinosarcoma, *see* carcinoma, in pleomorphic adenoma		
Cyst, extravasated	36	116
–, lymphoepithelial	36	119
–, retention	36	117
–, salivary duct	36	118

Cystadenocarcinoma, papillary 26   71, 72
Cystadenoma 16   29–31
–, mucinous 17   31
–, papillary 16   29, 30
Cystic lymphoid hyperplasia in AIDS 37   122–124

Dysgenetic polycystic disease 37   120

Infarction, salivary gland, *see* sialometaplasia, necrotizing

Küttner tumour, *see* sialadenitis, chronic sclerosing, of
  submandibular gland

Lesion, benign lymphoepithelial 35   114, 115
–, tumour-like 34   106–124
Lymphadenocarcinoma, sebaceous 26   –
Lymphadenoma, sebaceous 15   23
Lymphomas, malignant 32   101–103

Malignant mixed tumour, *see* carcinoma, in pleomorphic
  adenoma
Myoepithelioma 12   6, 7
–, malignant 28   80–83

Oncocytoma 14   17–19
Oncocytosis 35   107–109

Papilloma, ductal 16   24–28
–, intraductal 16   26
–, inverted ductal 16   24, 25

Salivary gland infarction, *see* sialometaplasia, necrotizing
Sialadenitis, chronic sclerosing, of submandibular gland 37   121
Sialadenoma papilliferum 16   27, 28
Sialadenosis 34   106
Sialometaplasia, necrotizing 35   110–113

Tumour, malignant mixed, *see* carcinoma, in pleomorphic
  adenoma
Tumours, secondary 33   104, 105
–, non-epithelial 31   98–100
–, unclassified 34   –

Warthin tumour 13   12–16

Unless otherwise stated, all the preparations shown in the photomicrographs reproduced on the following pages were stained with haematoxylin-eosin.

Acknowledgement. Figures 27 and 28 were made available by Dr. J. van der
Waal, Amsterdam, The Netherlands.

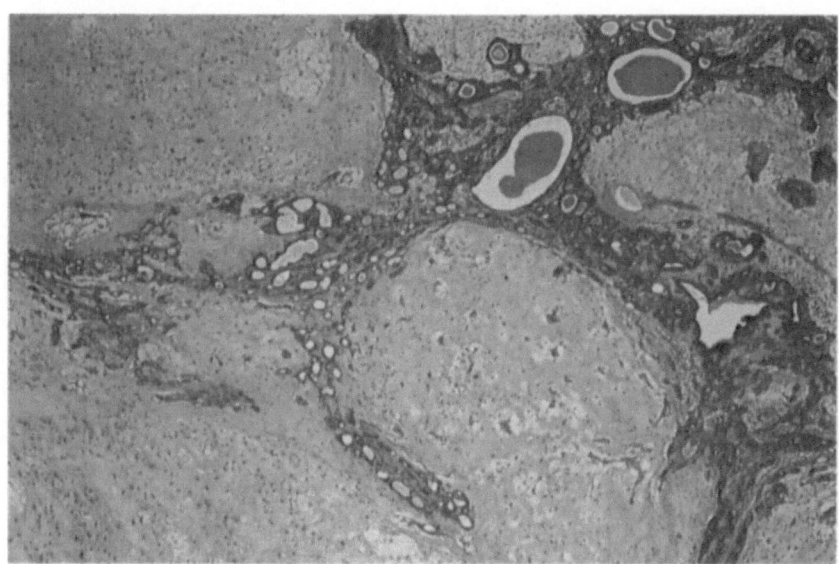

Fig. 1. *Pleomorphic adenoma*
Strands and sheets of epithelial cells with inclusion of ducts and myxochondroid areas

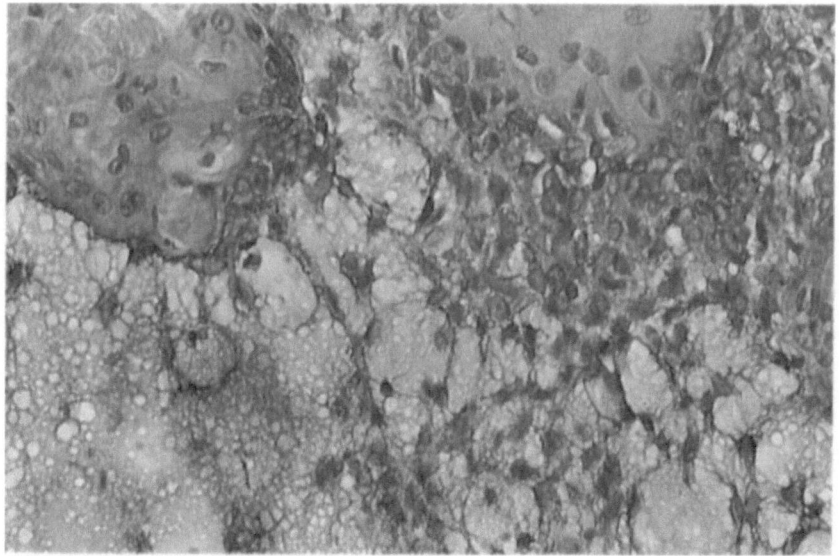

Fig. 2. *Pleomorphic adenoma*
Solid areas with squamous metaplasia *(upper field)*. Myoepithelial cells appear to melt into the myxoid background *(lower field)*. Astra blue

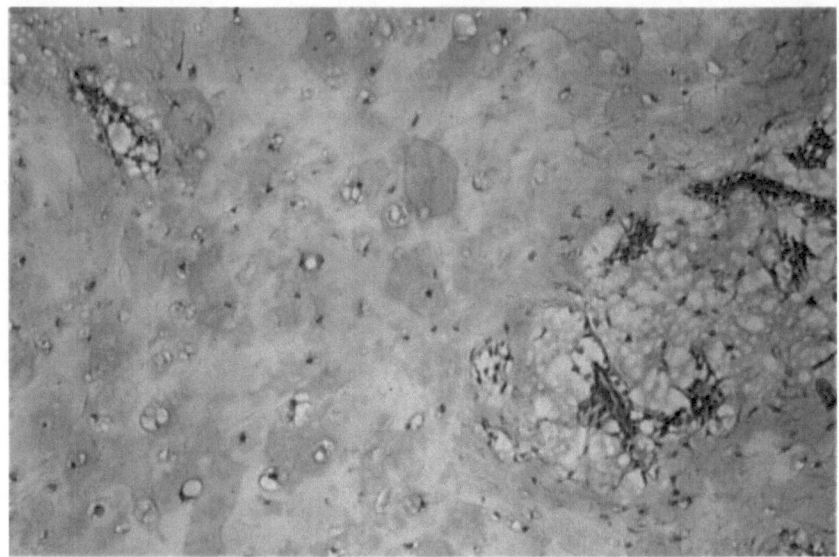

Fig. 3. *Pleomorphic adenoma*
Stroma-rich area with spindle-shaped myoepithelial cells in myxochondroid
stroma. Astra blue

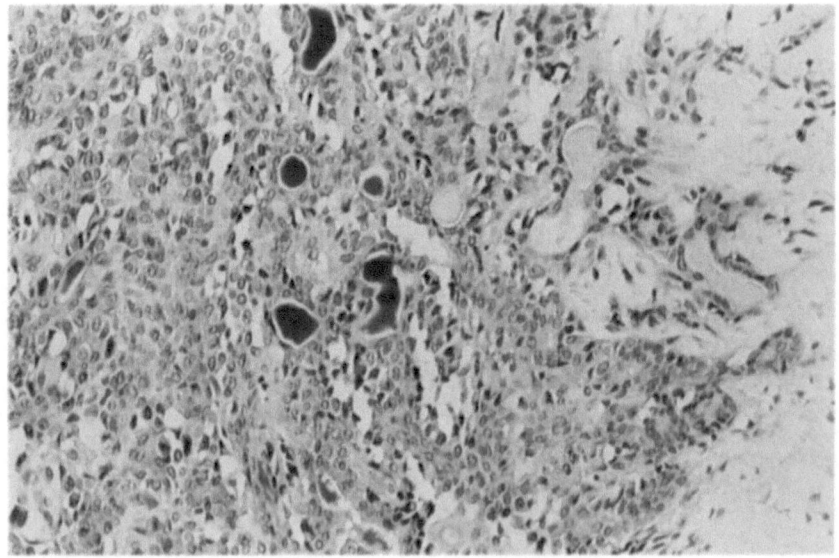

Fig. 4. *Pleomorphic adenoma*
Cell-rich variant with inclusion of duct-like structures. Masson-Goldner

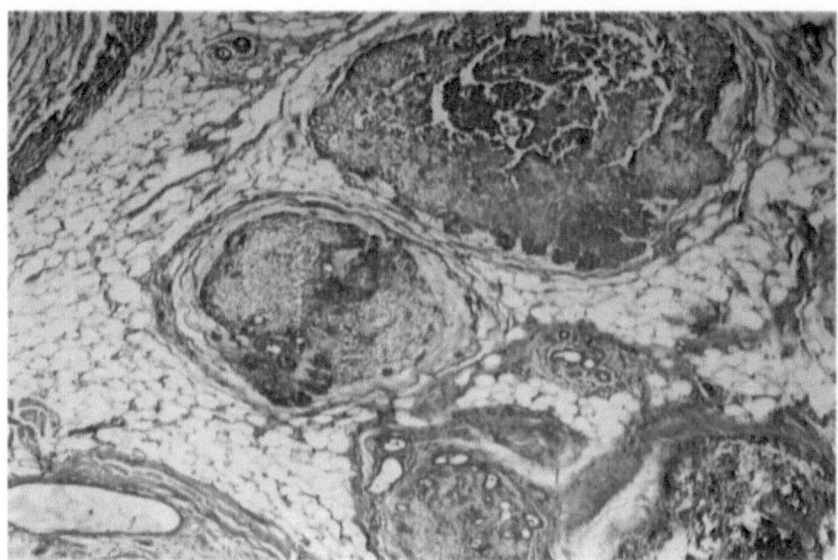

Fig. 5. *Pleomorphic adenoma*
Multifocal extension into the surrounding fatty tissue due to tumour implantation after capsule rupture during removal

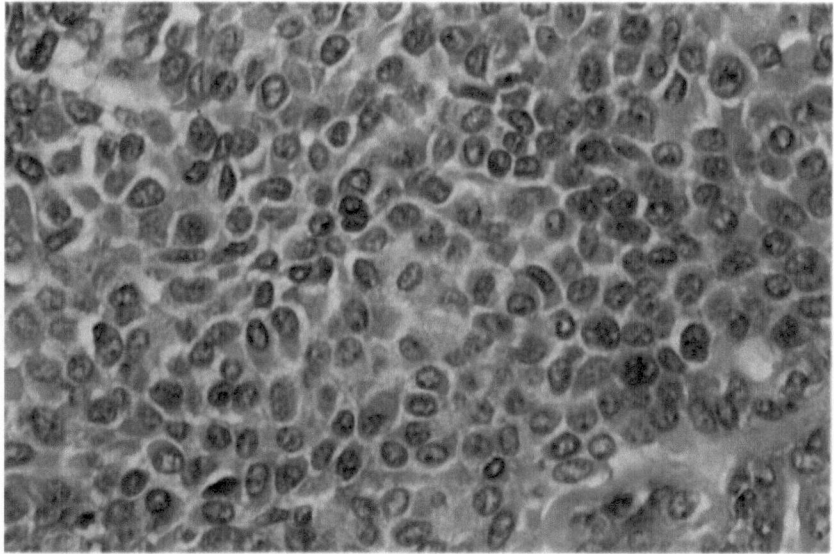

Fig. 6. *Myoepithelioma*
Solid pattern with plasmacytoid (hyaline) cells without duct-like structures

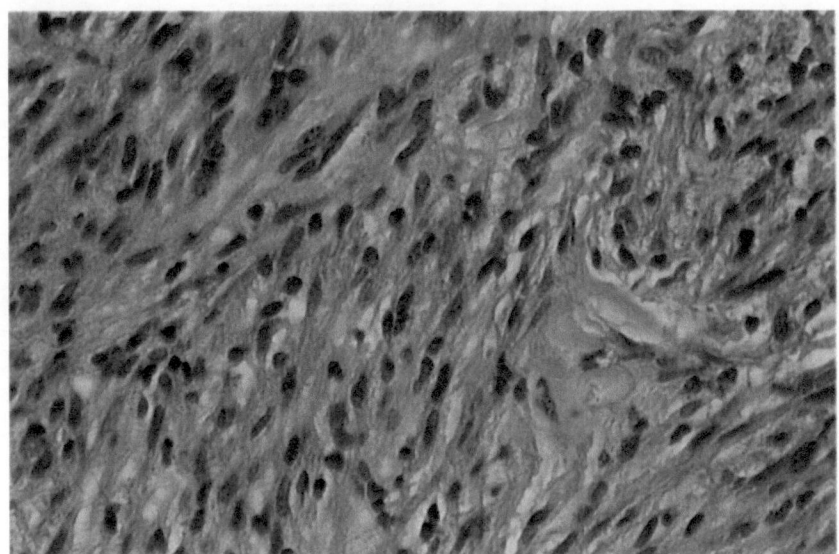

Fig. 7. *Myoepithelioma*
Solid pattern with spindle-shaped cells. No duct-like structures

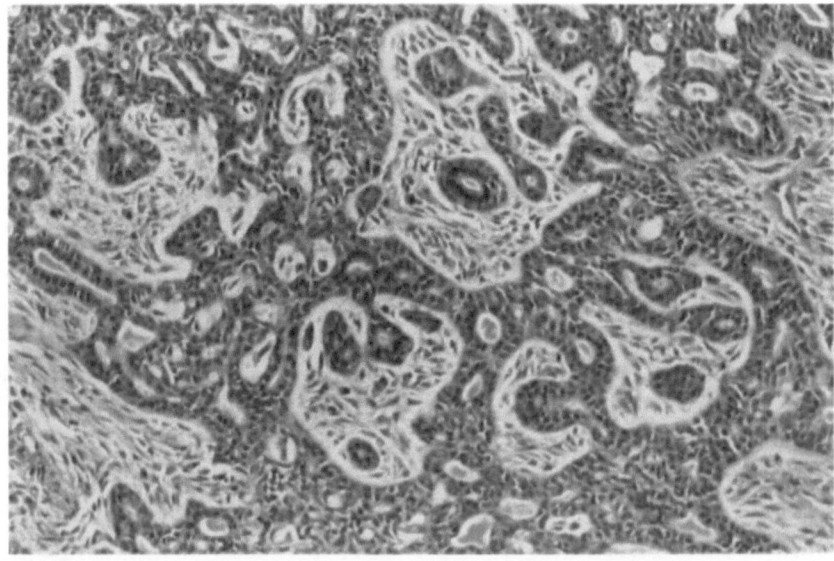

Fig. 8. *Basal cell adenoma*
Trabecular and tubular variant. Absence of mucoid stromal component

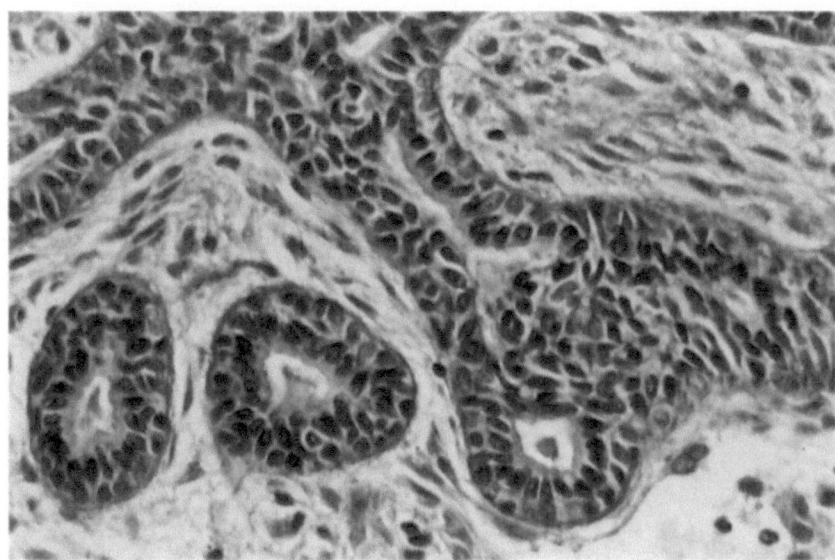

Fig. 9. *Basal cell adenoma*
Predominantly tubular variant with distinct basement membrane-like material
on the outside. Periodic acid-Schiff

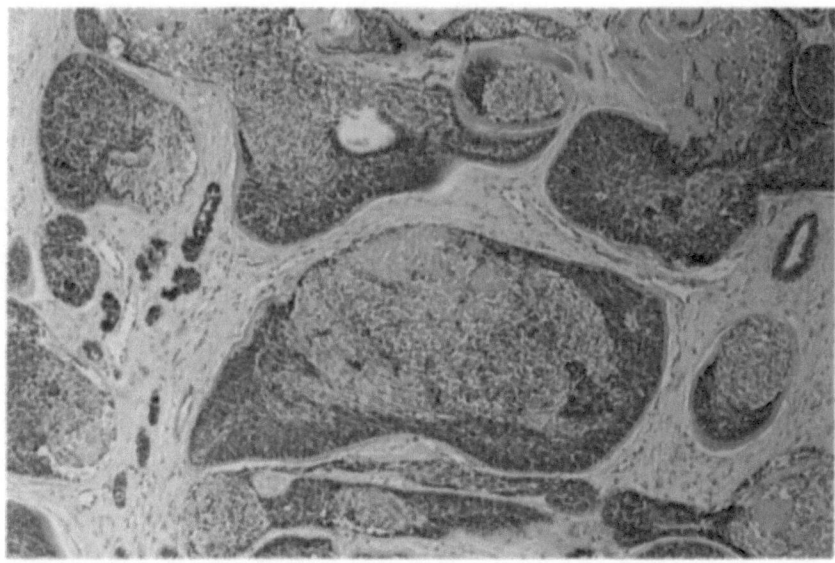

Fig. 10. *Basal cell adenoma*
Membranous variant (dermal anlage type) with multifocal development of
microadenomas

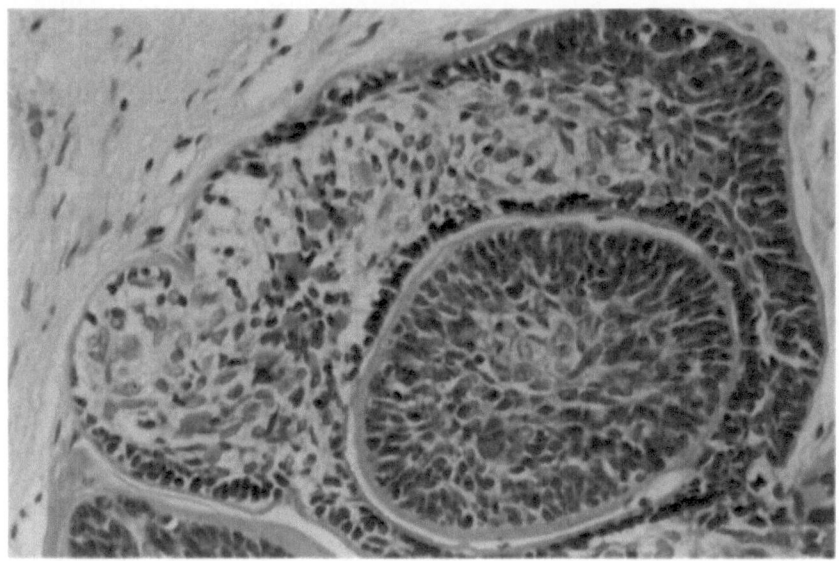

Fig. 11. *Basal cell adenoma*
Membranous variant with palisading of peripheral cells, hyaline basal membrane and intercellular deposits

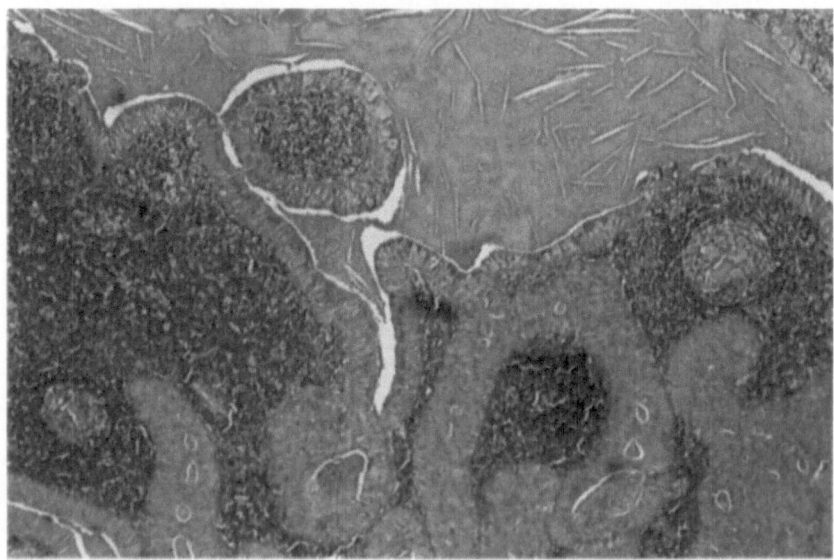

Fig. 12. *Warthin tumour*
Glandular oncocytic epithelium in papillary-cystic arrangements with intervening lymphoid tissue

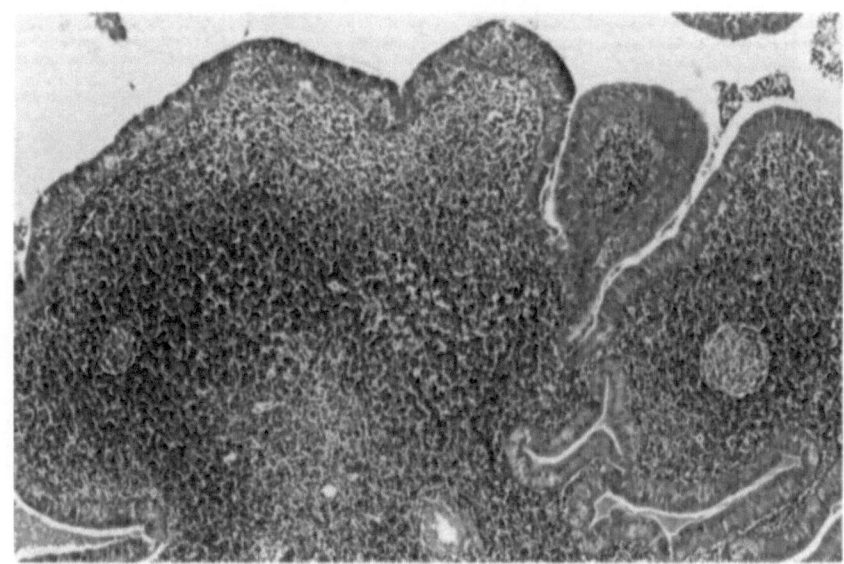

Fig. 13. *Warthin tumour*
Predominance of lymphoid stromal component

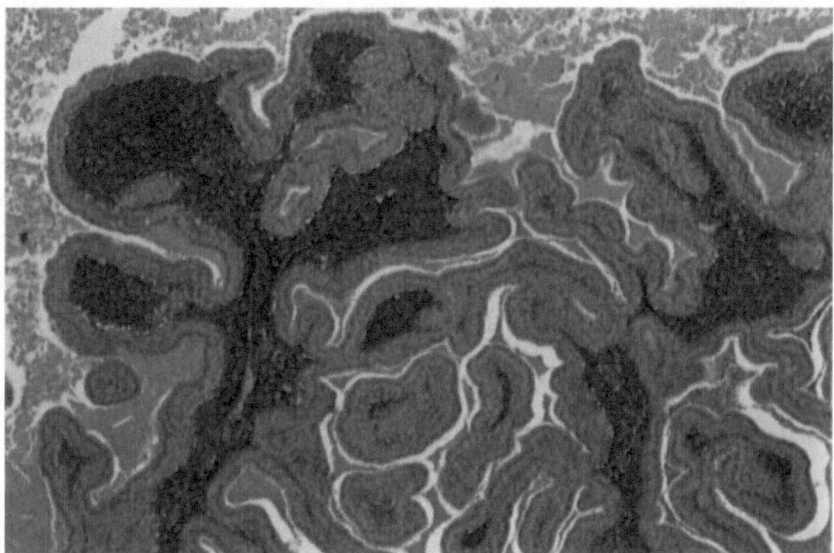

Fig. 14. *Warthin tumour*
Predominance of oncocytic cells and small lymphoid stromal areas

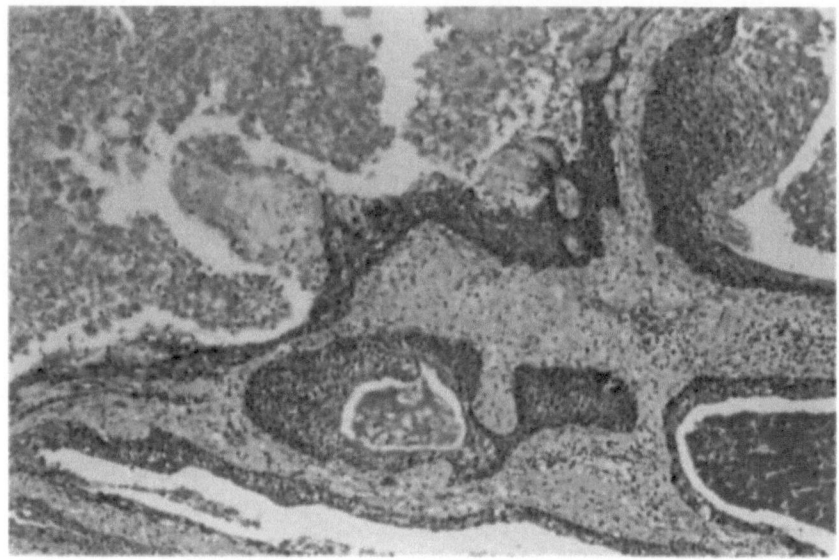

Fig. 15. *Warthin tumour*
Metaplastic (infected or infarcted) variant with squamous metaplasia and regressive stromal changes

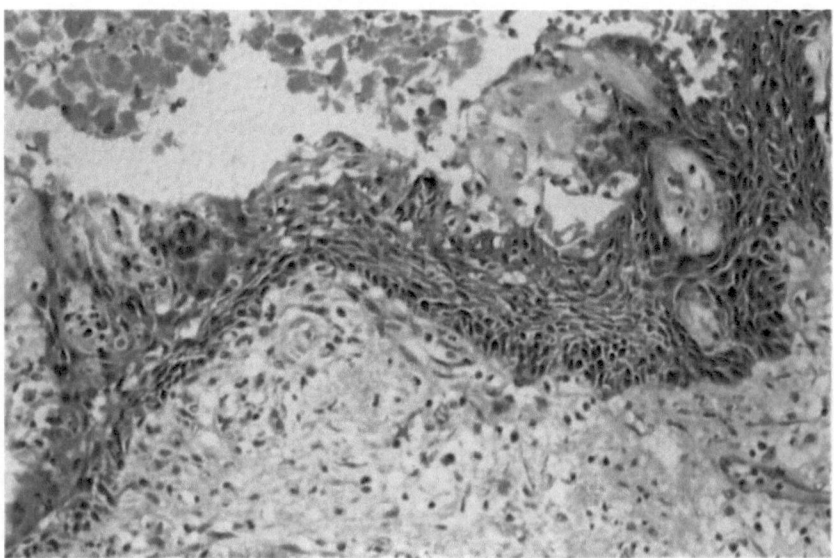

Fig. 16. *Warthin tumour*
Metaplastic variant with squamous metaplasia

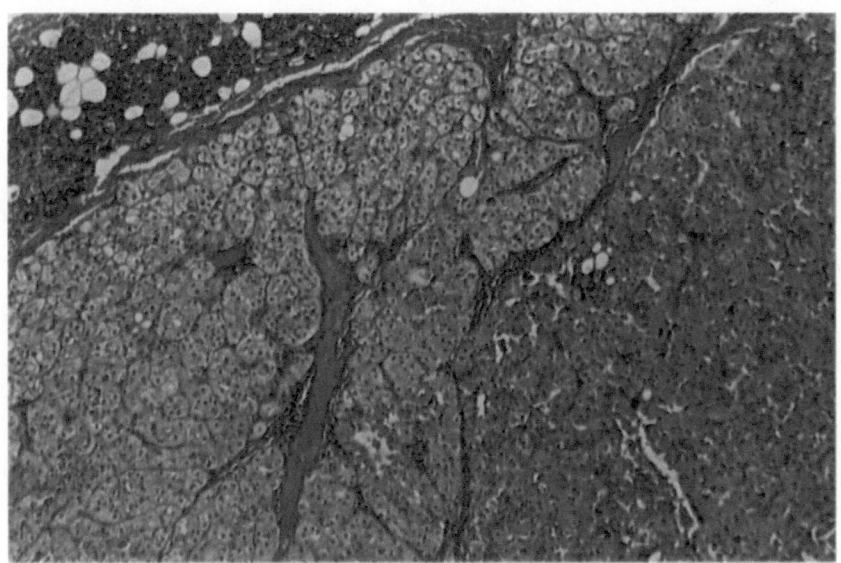

Fig. 17. *Oncocytoma*
Solid sheets of eosinophilic cells with some clear cell areas and surrounded by a
thin capsule

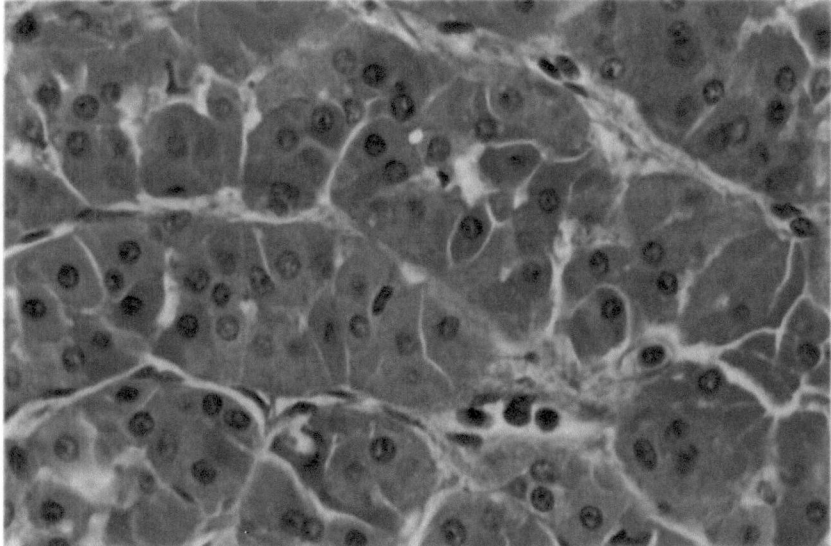

Fig. 18. *Oncocytoma*
Typical oncocytic cells with intensely eosinophilic granular cytoplasm and small
nuclei

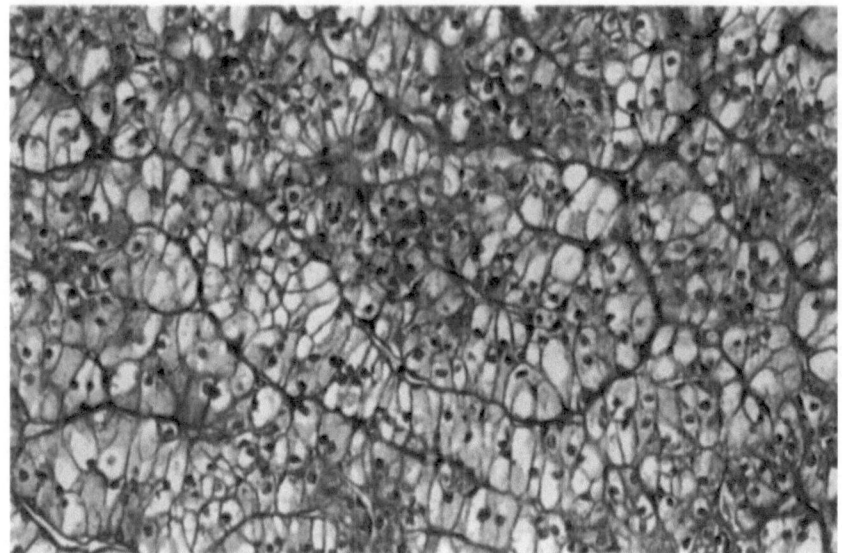

Fig. 19. *Oncocytoma*
Clear cell variant. Periodic acid-Schiff

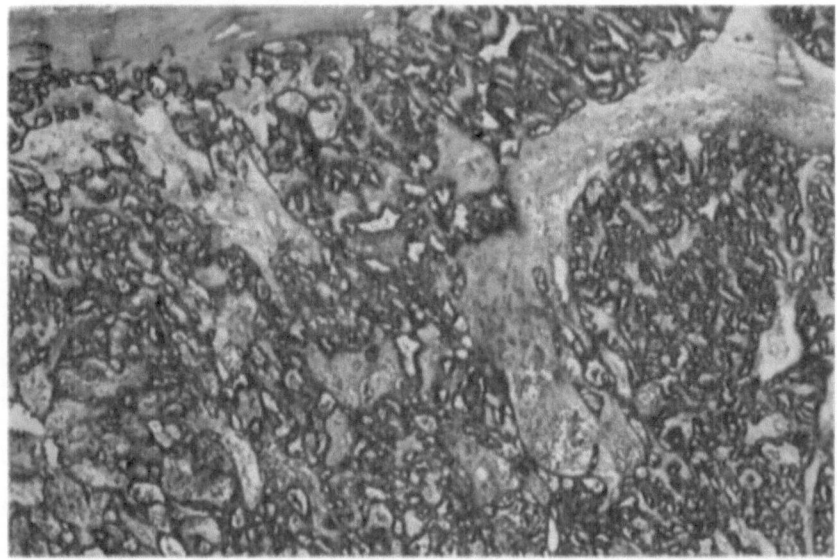

Fig. 20. *Canalicular adenoma*
Anastomosing strands with a beading pattern

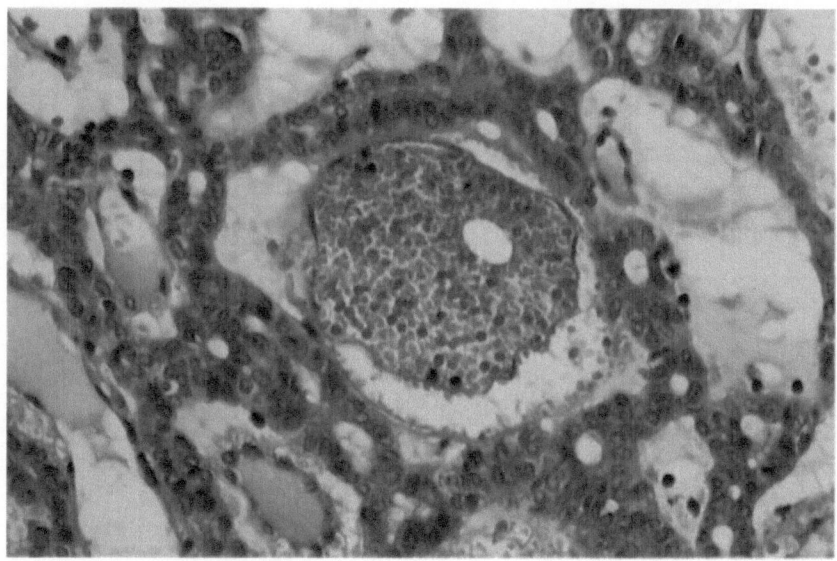

Fig. 21. *Canalicular adenoma*
Loose, highly vascular stroma

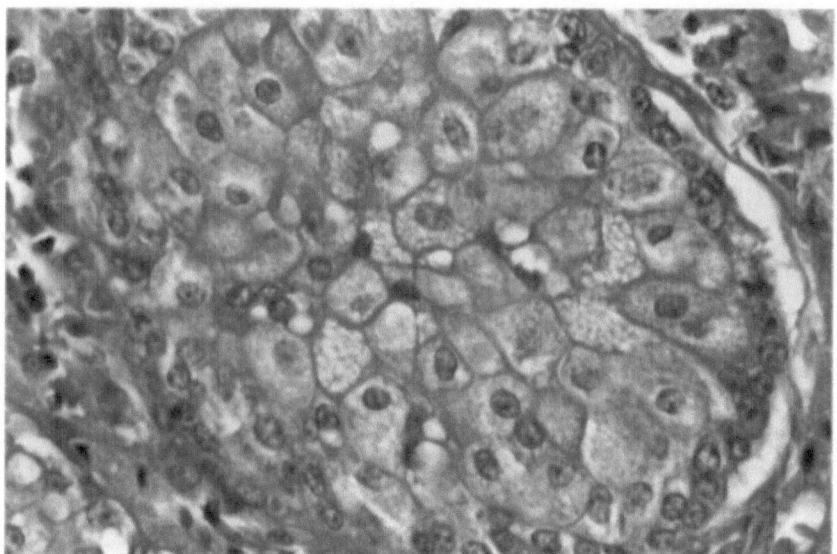

Fig. 22. *Sebaceous adenoma*
Nests of sebaceous cells in a lobular arrangement

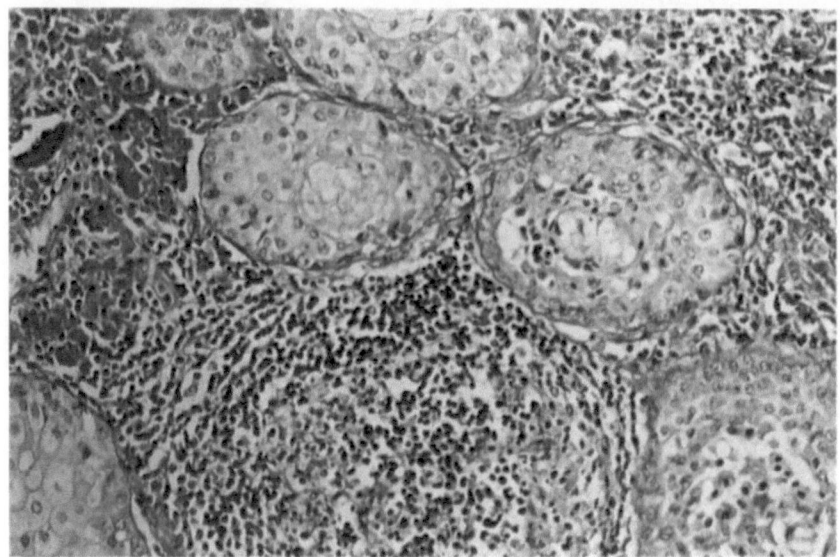

Fig. 23. *Sebaceous lymphadenoma*
Glandular configuration of sebaceous cells lying in a lymphoid stroma. Periodic
acid-Schiff

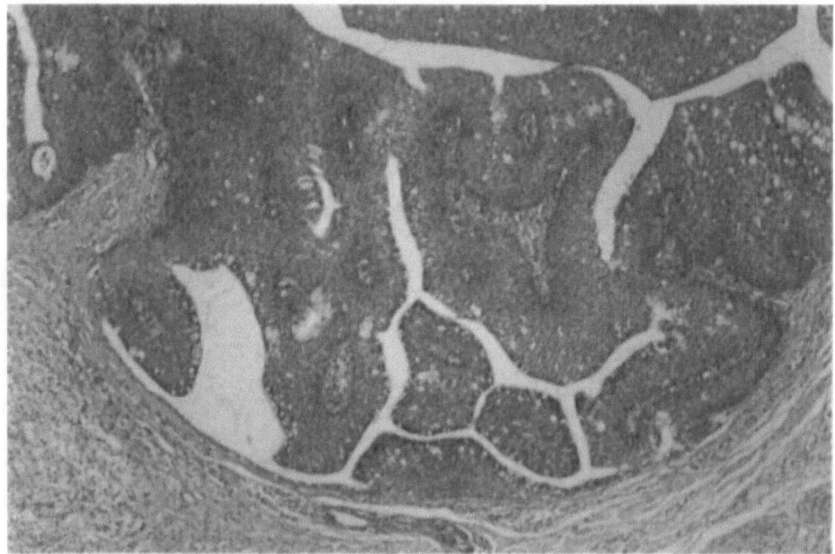

Fig. 24. *Inverted ductal papilloma*
Extension of squamous epithelial cells into the surrounding tissue

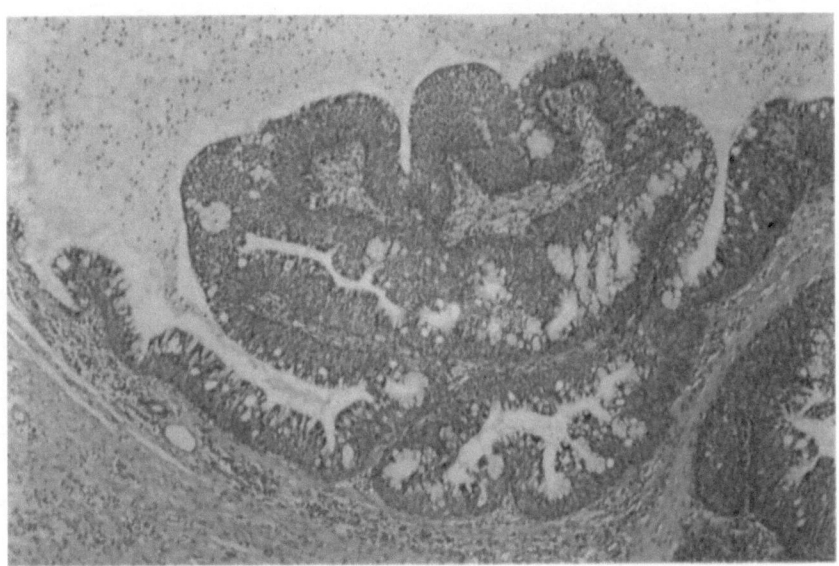

Fig. 25. *Inverted ductal papilloma*
Some mucous cells between the epithelial cells

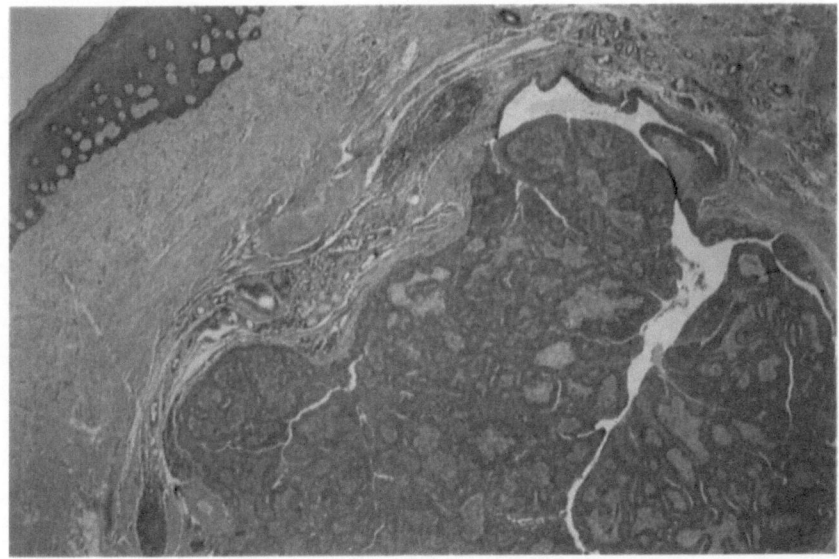

Fig. 26. *Intraductal papilloma*
Papillary intraductal projections

64

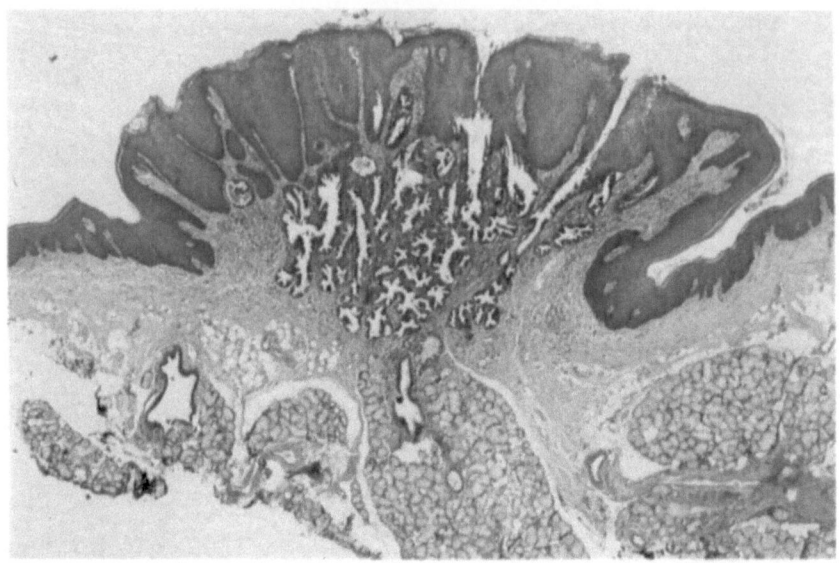

Fig. 27. *Sialadenoma papilliferum*
Duct-like structures in continuity with the surface of the oral mucosa

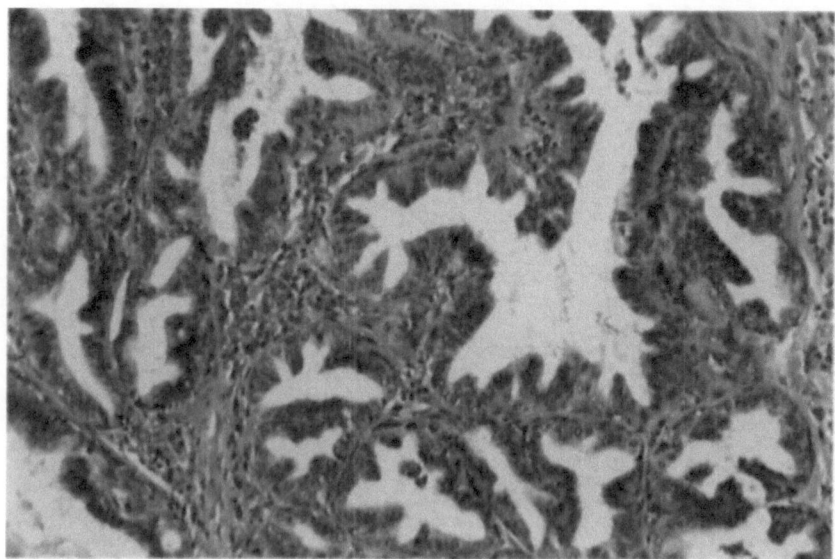

Fig. 28. *Sialadenoma papilliferum*
Small papillary projections into microcysts

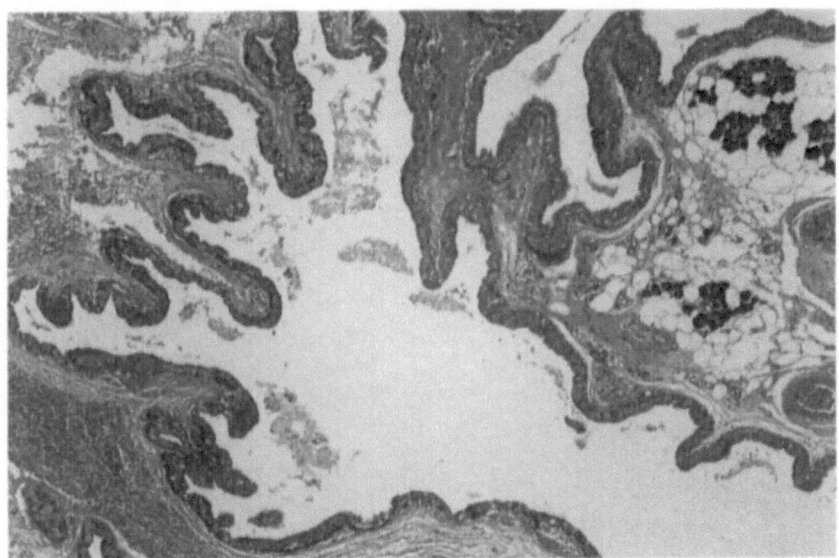

Fig. 29. *Papillary cystadenoma*
Multicystic areas with papillary projections

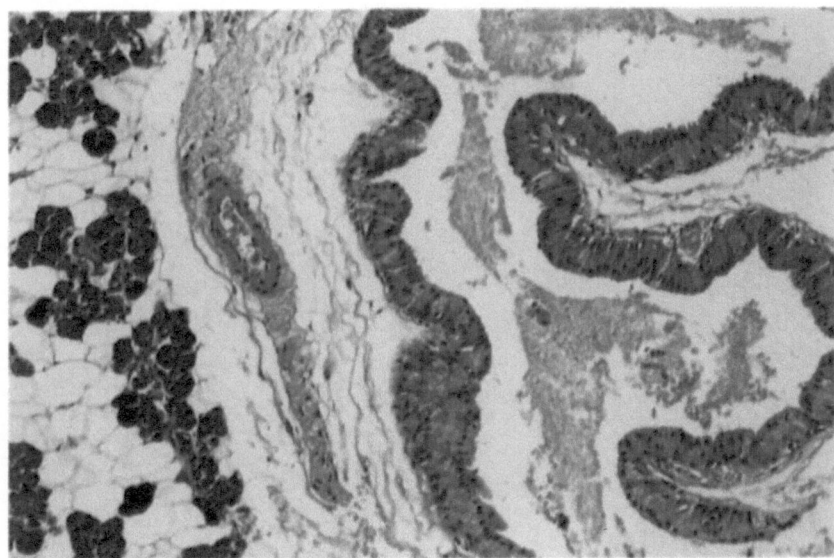

Fig. 30 *Papillary cystadenoma*
Oncocytic cells line cystic spaces

66

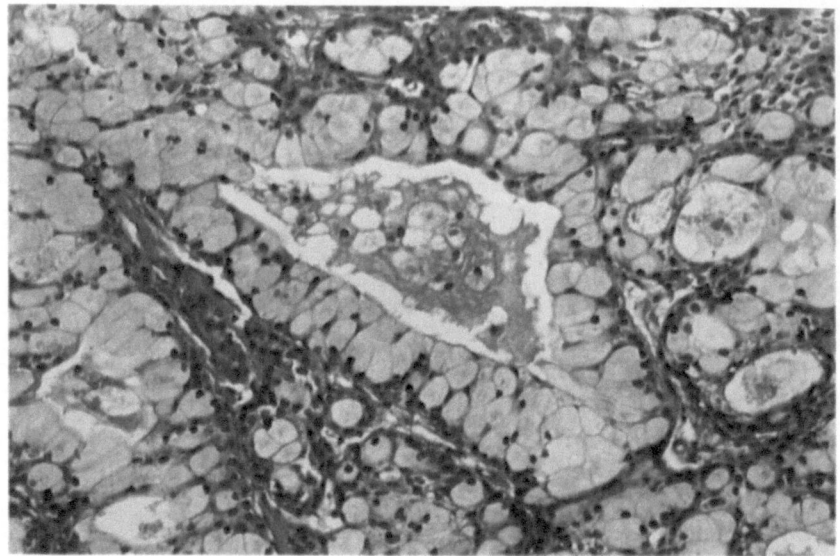

Fig. 31. *Mucinous cystadenoma*
Cystic spaces lined by mucus-producing cells

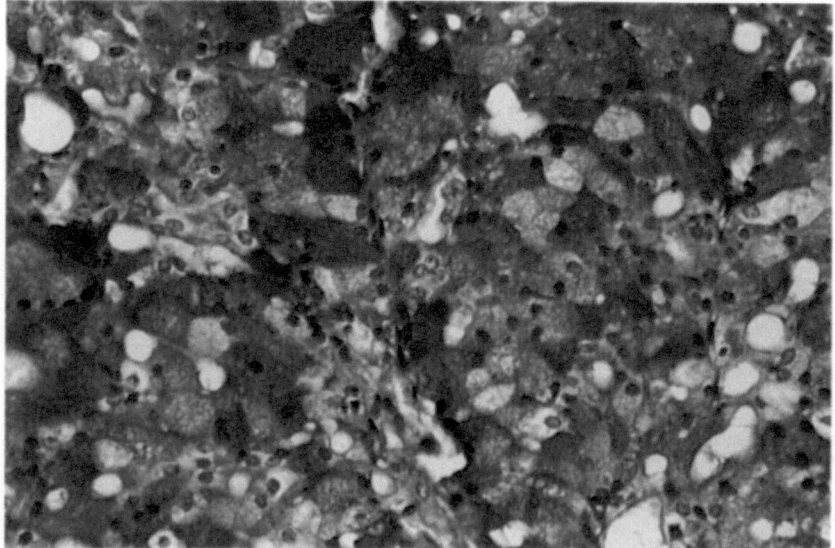

Fig. 32. *Acinic cell carcinoma*
Acinic tumour cells with periodic acid-Schiff-positive cytoplasmic granules.

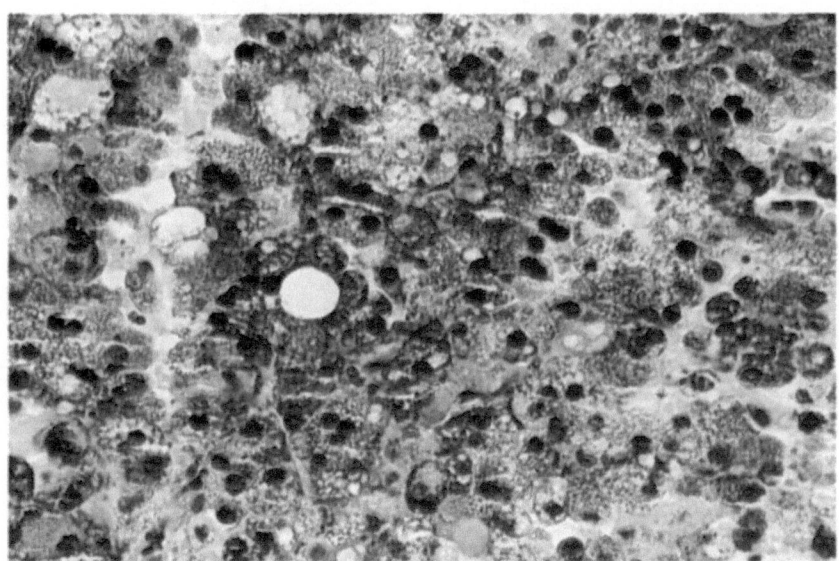

Fig. 33. *Acinic cell carcinoma*
Acinic tumour cells with positive amylase reaction. Immunocytochemical
peroxidase-antiperoxidase method

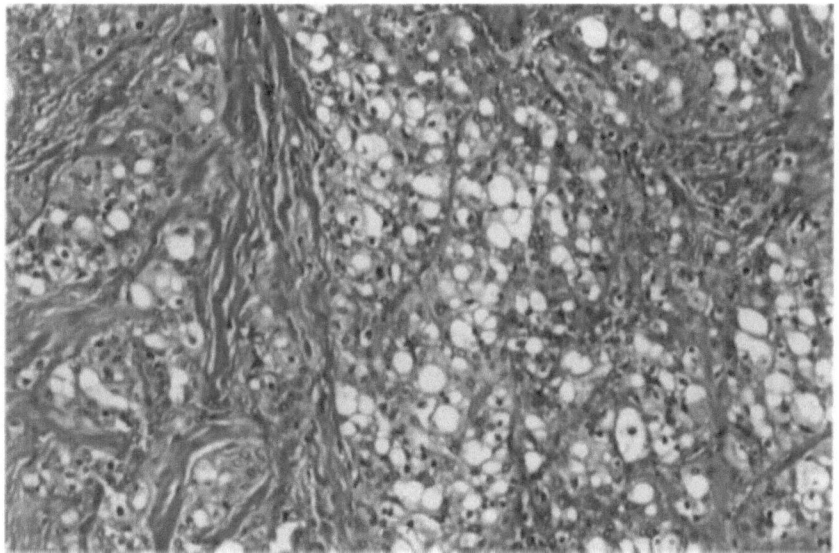

Fig. 34. *Acinic cell carcinoma*
Clear cell variant

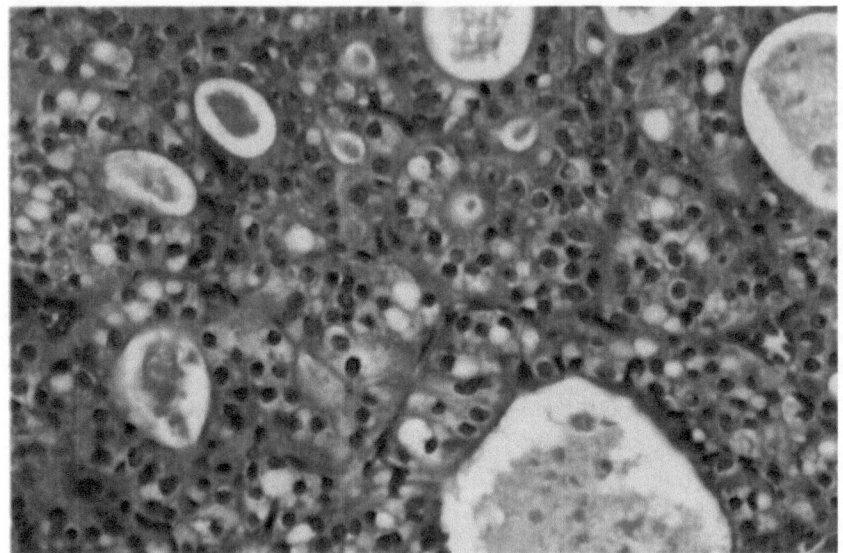

Fig. 35. *Acinic cell carcinoma*
Intercalated duct-like cell arrangements

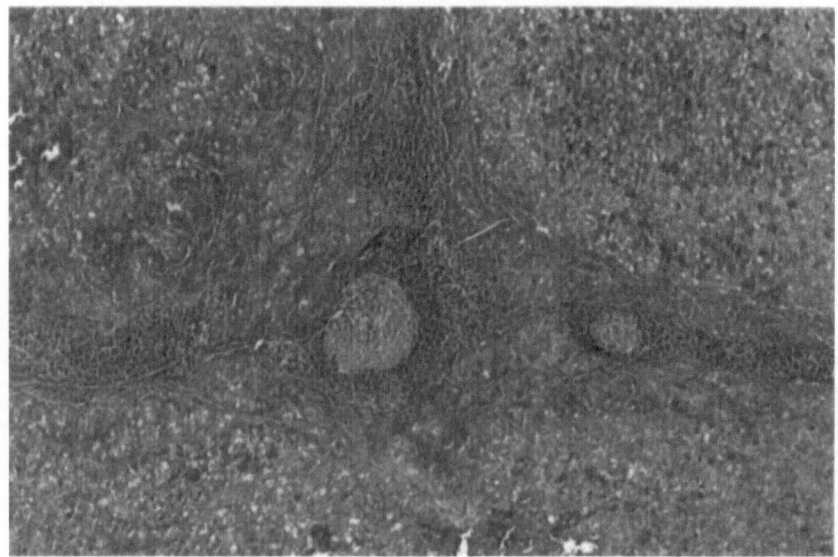

Fig. 36. *Acinic cell carcinoma*
Solid pattern with lymphoid stromal component

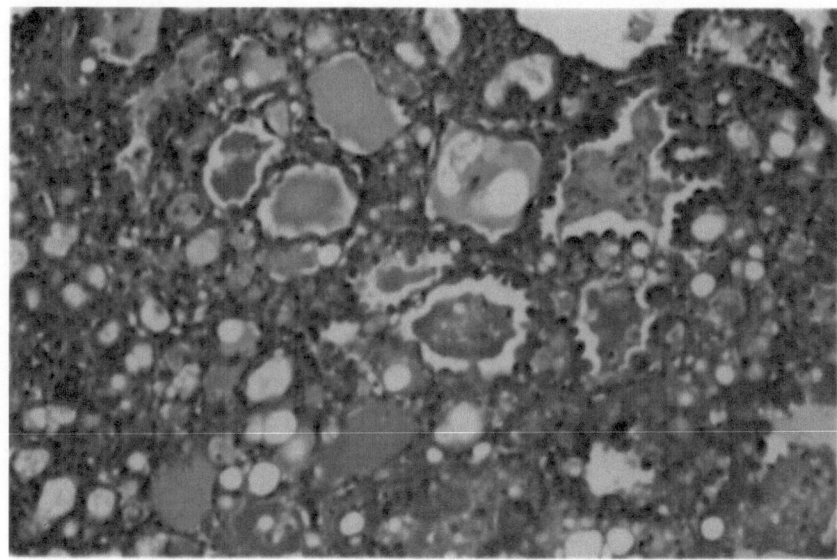

Fig. 37. *Acinic cell carcinoma*
Microcystic pattern

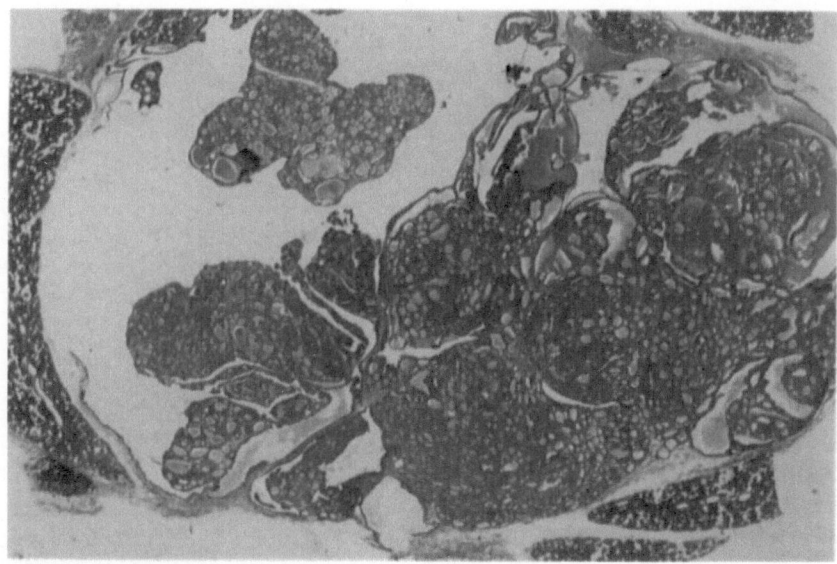

Fig. 38. *Acinic cell carcinoma*
Papillary-cystic pattern

70

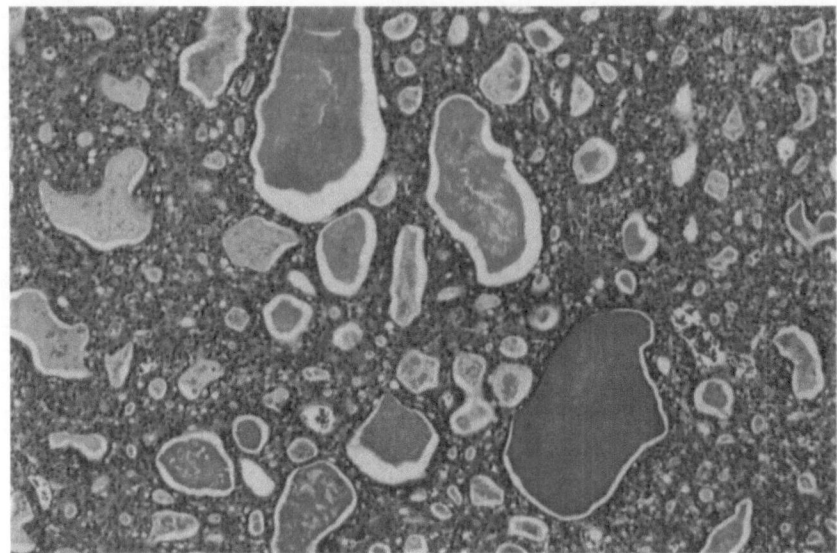

Fig. 39. *Acinic cell carcinoma*
Follicular (thyroid-like) pattern

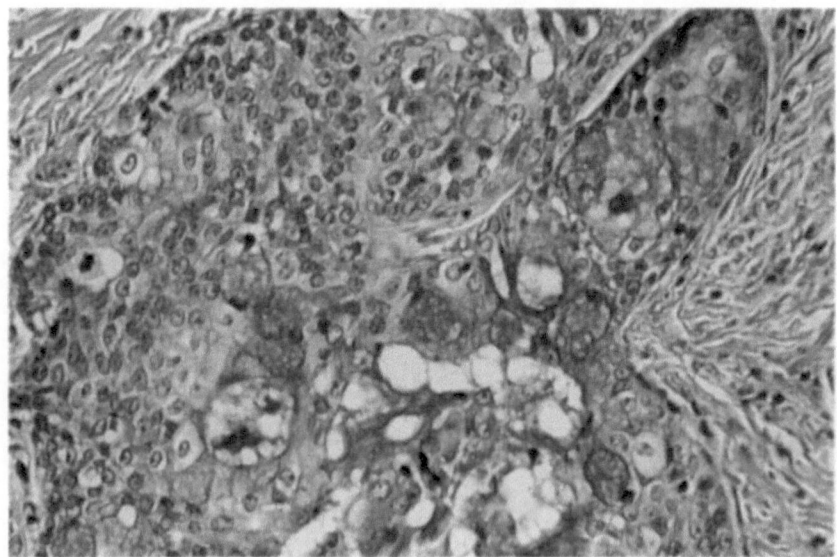

Fig. 40. *Mucoepidermoid carcinoma*
Biphasic pattern with squamous cells and mucus-producing cells. Periodic acid-
Schiff

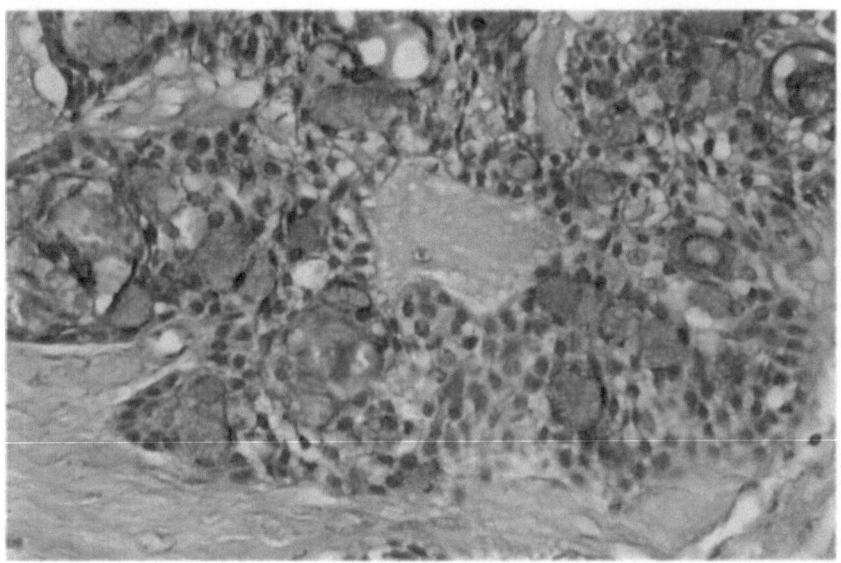

Fig. 41. *Mucoepidermoid carcinoma*
Goblet-like cells between solid epidermoid cell formations. Astra blue

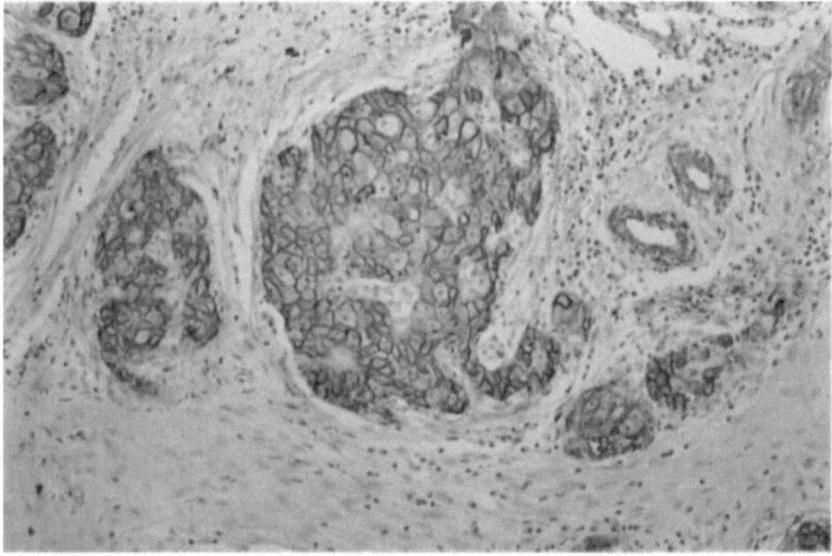

Fig. 42. *Mucoepidermoid carcinoma*
Strong epithelial membrane antigen reaction in the epidermoid cells. Immunocytochemical peroxidase-antiperoxidase method

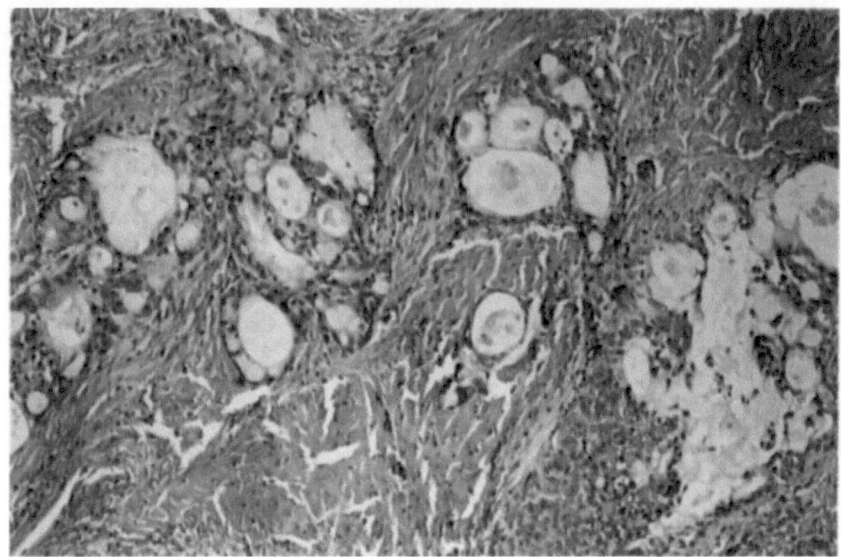

Fig. 43. *Mucoepidermoid carcinoma*
Invasive growth with moderate stromal reaction

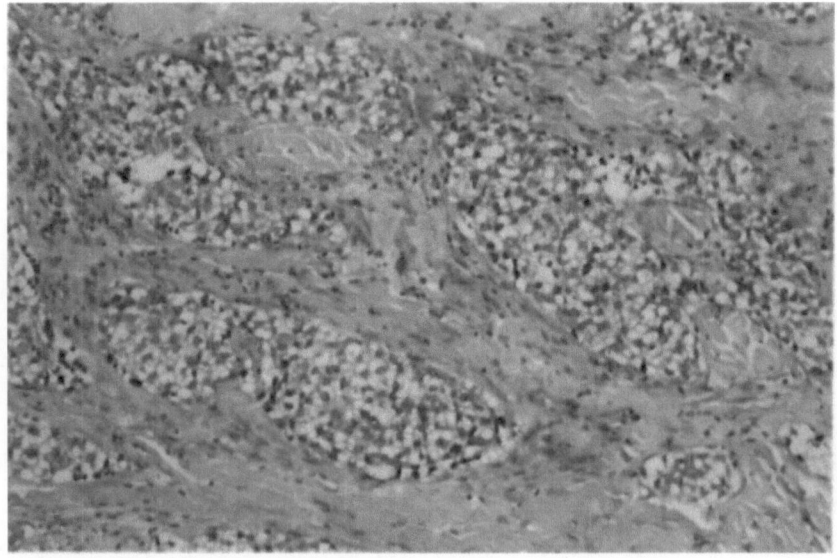

Fig. 44. *Mucoepidermoid carcinoma*
Clear cell variant

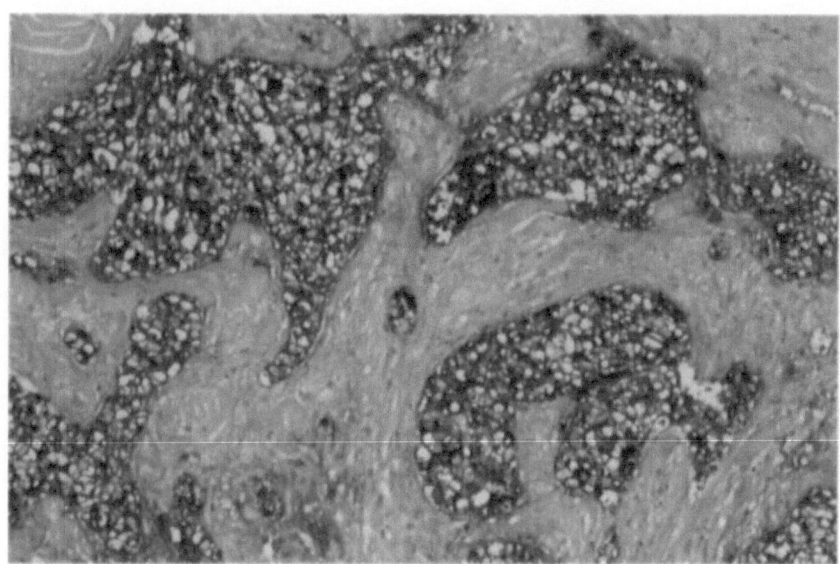

Fig. 45. *Mucoepidermoid carcinoma*
Clear cell variant with strong periodic acid-Schiff reaction

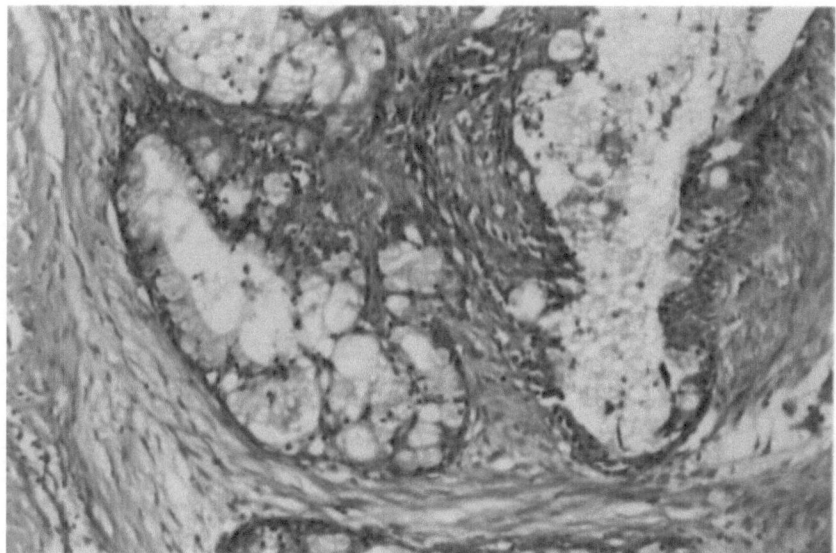

Fig. 46. *Mucoepidermoid carcinoma*
Well-differentiated type (low-grade tumour) with predominance of cystic
spaces and mucus-producing cells

74

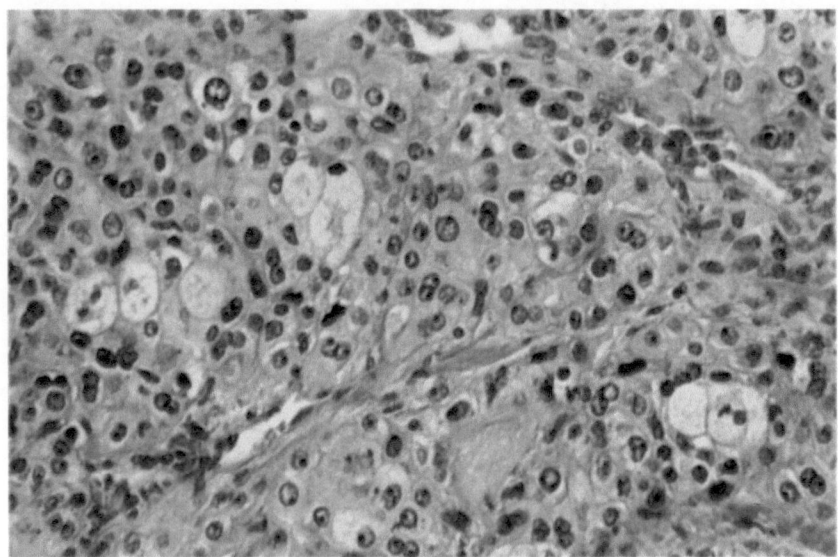

Fig. 47. *Mucoepidermoid carcinoma*
Poorly differentiated type (high-grade tumour) with predominance of intermediate cells and only isolated mucus-producing cells

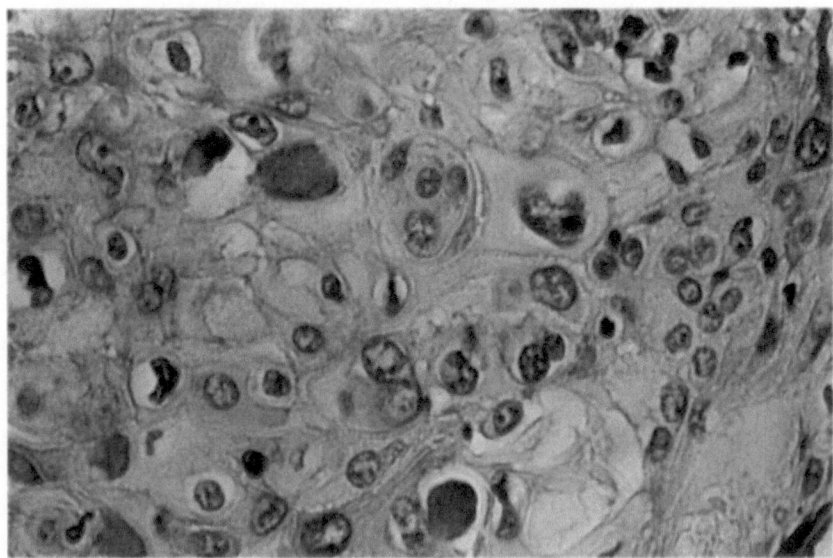

Fig. 48. *Mucoepidermoid carcinoma*
Poorly differentiated type with isolated mucus-producing cells. Periodic acid-
Schiff

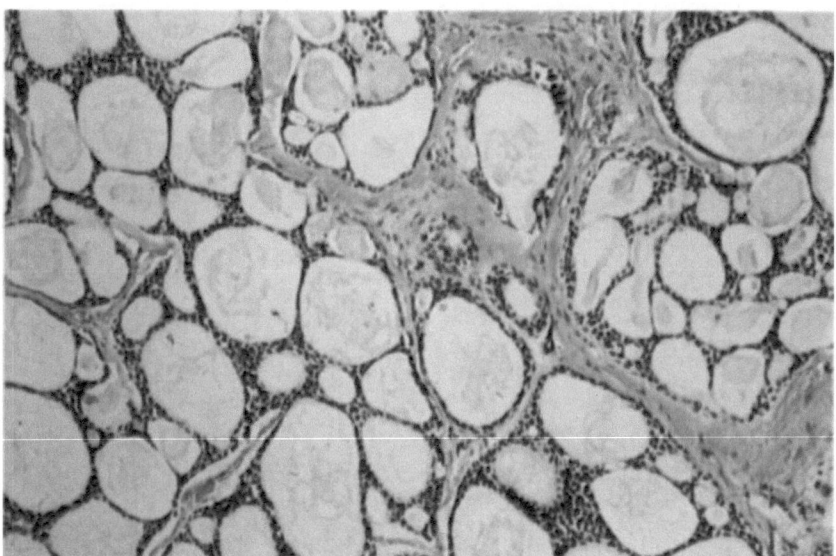

Fig. 49. *Adenoid cystic carcinoma*
Glandular (cribriform) type

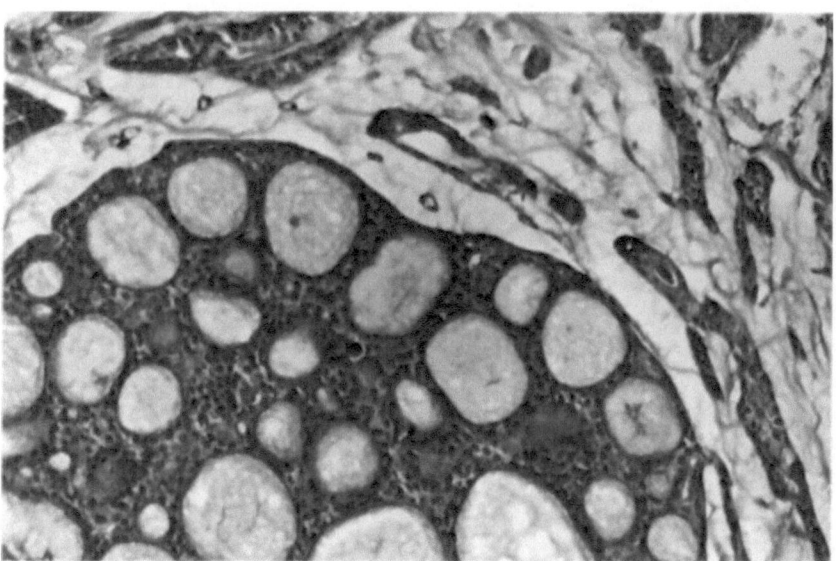

Fig. 50. *Adenoid cystic carcinoma*
Glandular type with Swiss-cheese pseudocysts. Periodic acid-Schiff

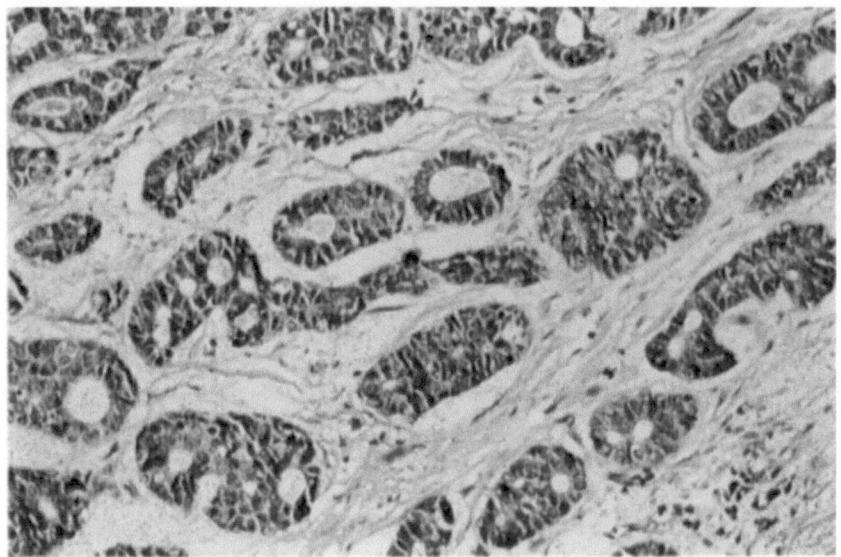

Fig. 51. *Adenoid cystic carcinoma*
Tubular type

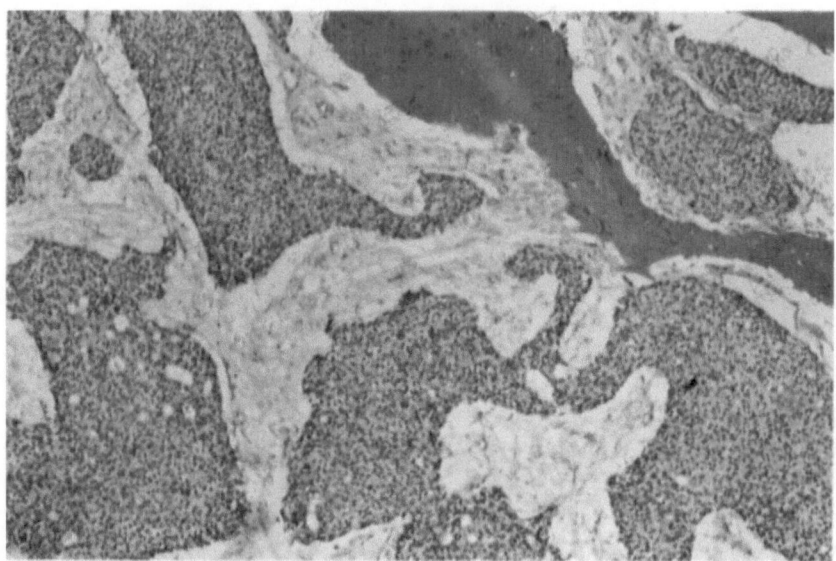

Fig. 52. *Adenoid cystic carcinoma*
Solid type with intraosseous growth

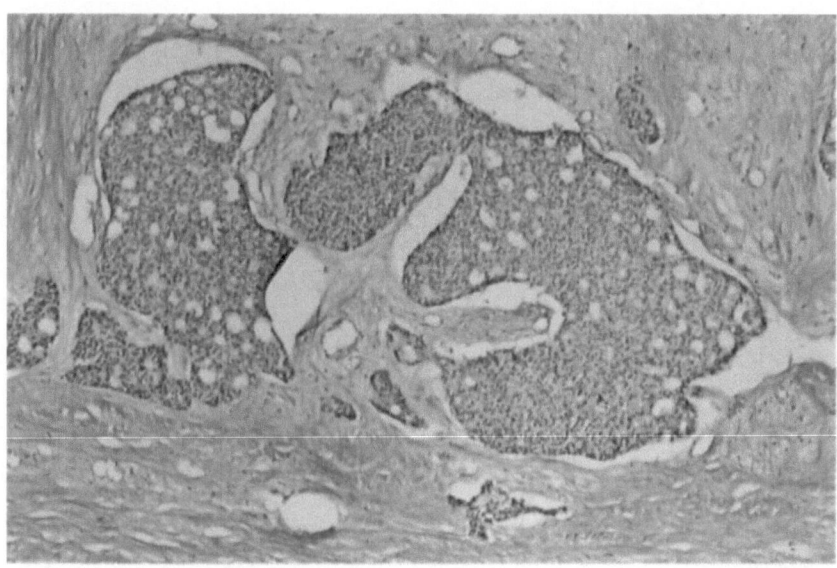

Fig. 53. *Adenoid cystic carcinoma*
Solid type with a few gland-like spaces and intravascular spread. No stromal reaction

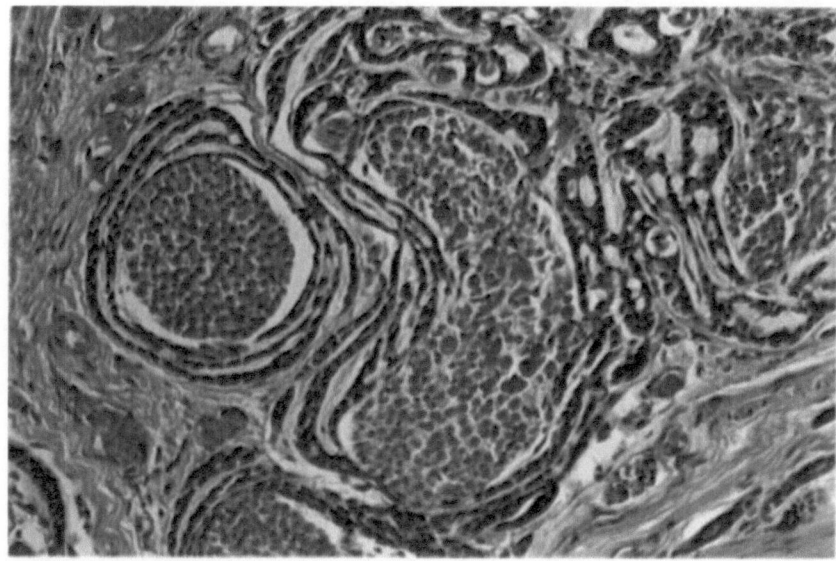

Fig. 54. *Adenoid cystic carcinoma*
Perineural infiltration

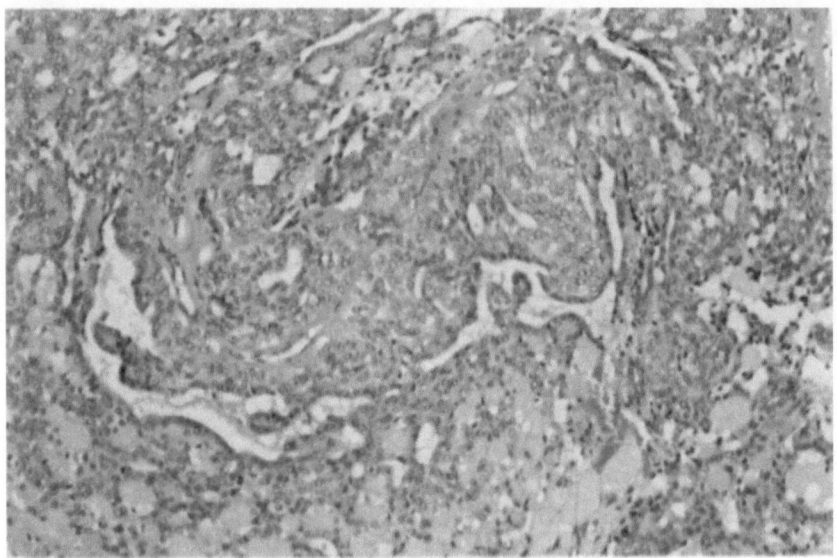

Fig. 55. *Polymorphous low-grade adenocarcinoma*
Pale glandular nests with duct-like structures

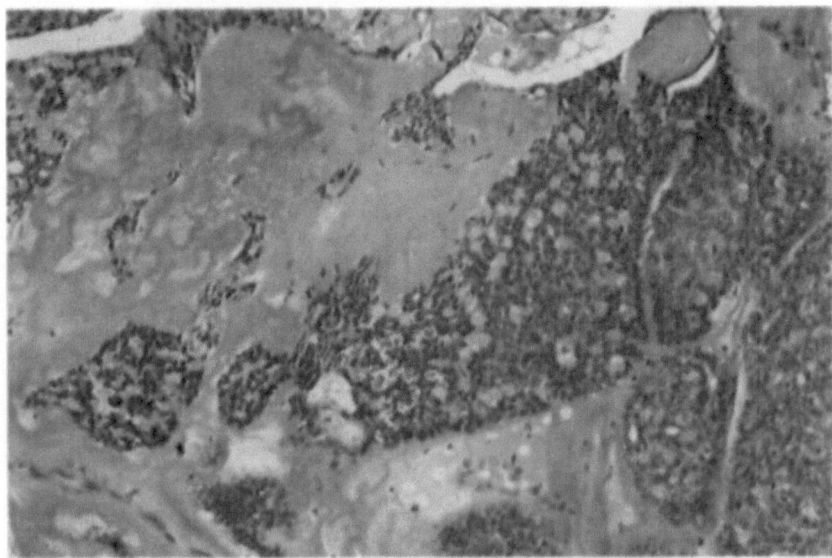

Fig. 56. *Polymorphous low-grade adenocarcinoma*
Cribriform-like areas with hyalinized stromal component

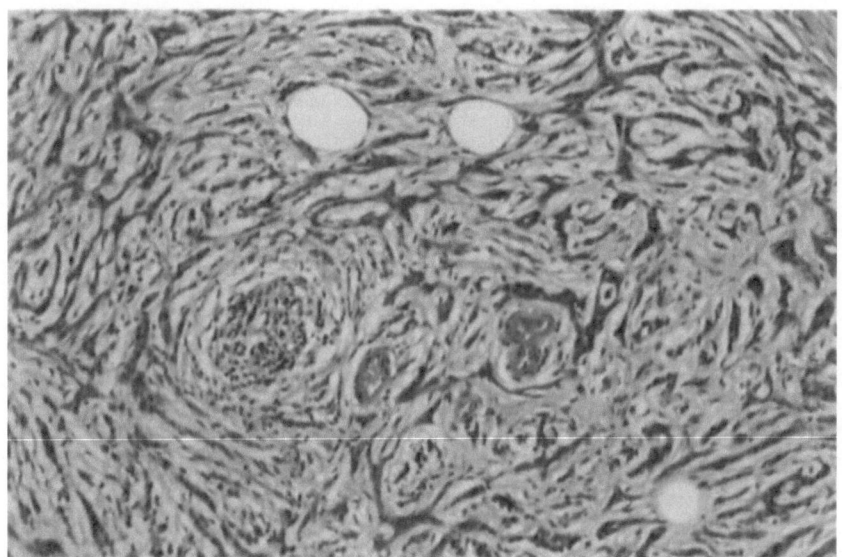

Fig. 57. *Polymorphous low-grade adenocarcinoma*
Formation of concentric whorls

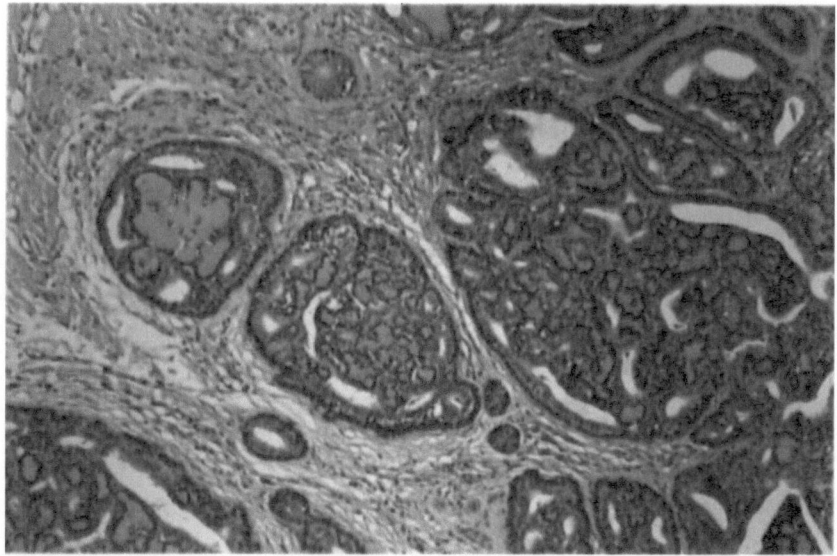

Fig. 58. *Polymorphous low-grade adenocarcinoma*
Papillary-cystic formations

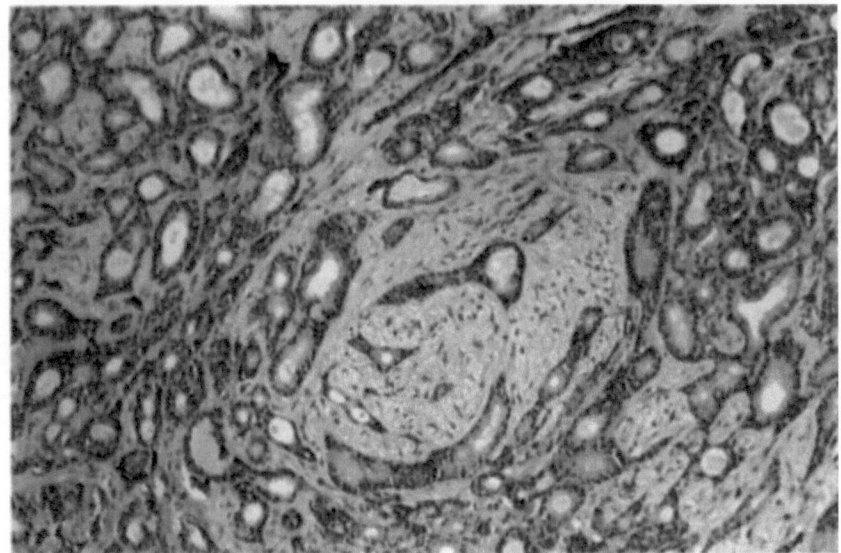

Fig. 59. *Polymorphous low-grade adenocarcinoma*
Tubular pattern

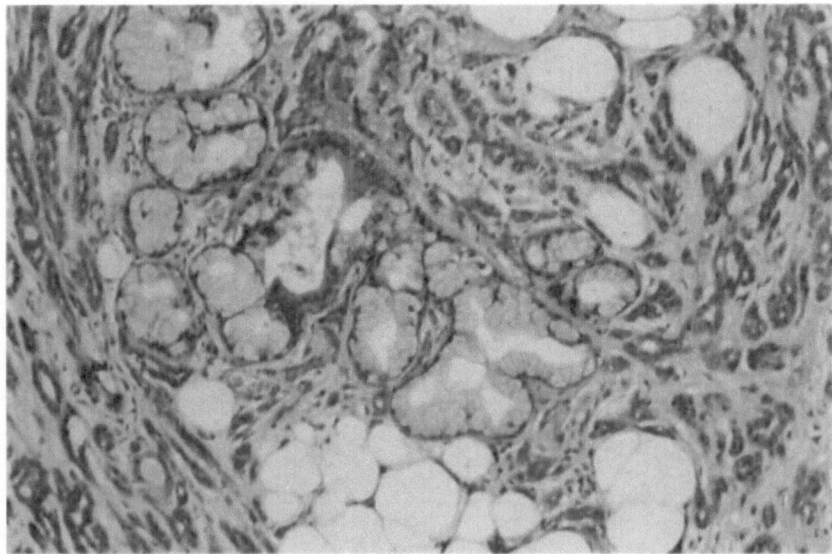

Fig. 60. *Polymorphous low-grade adenocarcinoma*
Invasion of the surrounding glandular tissue

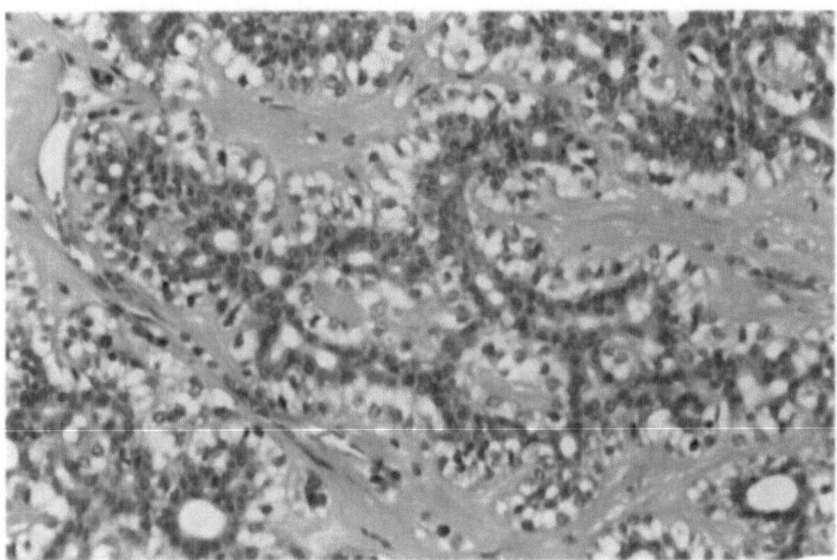

Fig. 61. *Epithelial-myoepithelial carcinoma*
Inner layer of dark duct lining cells and outer layer of clear myoepithelial cells .

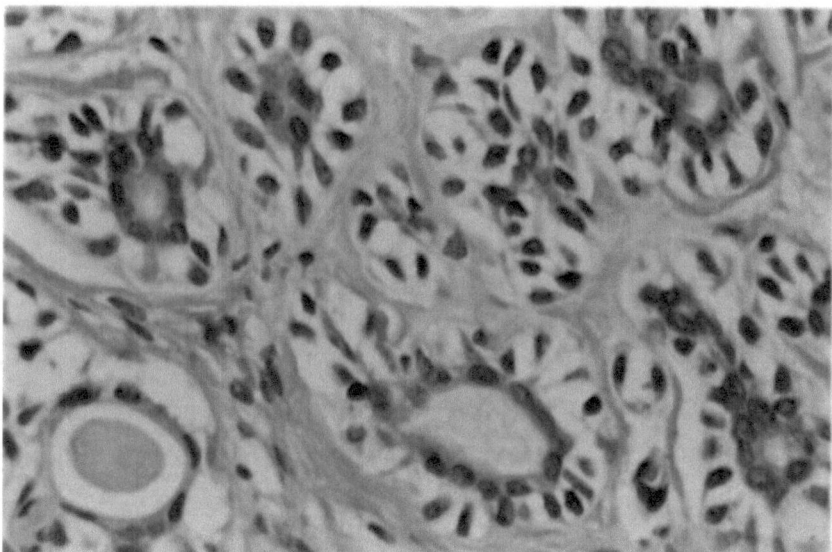

Fig. 62. *Epithelial-myoepithelial carcinoma*
Ducts with double layer of two cell types

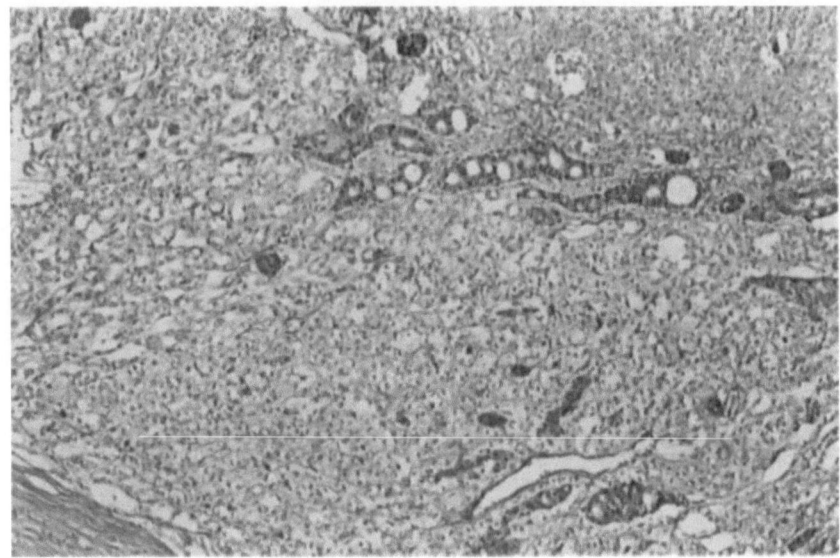

Fig. 63. *Epithelial-myoepithelial carcinoma*
Predominance of clear myoepithelial cells

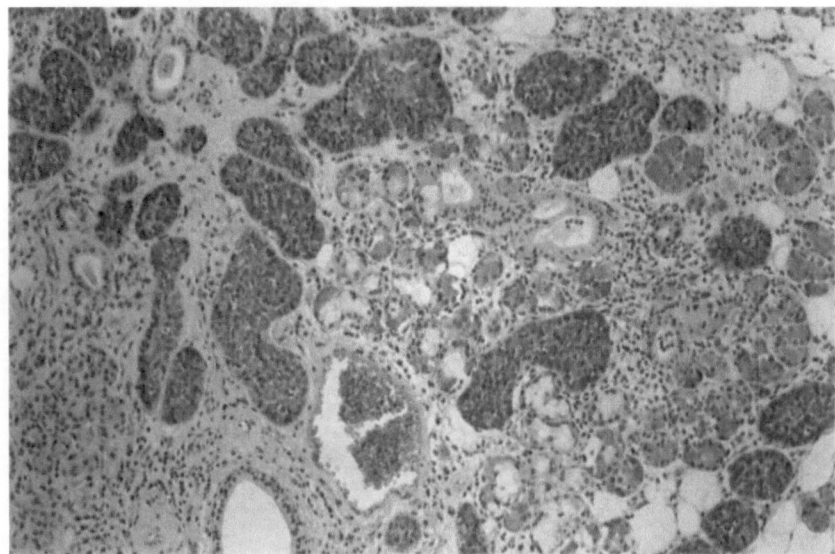

Fig. 64. *Basal cell adenocarcinoma*
Infiltration into the parotid gland parenchyma

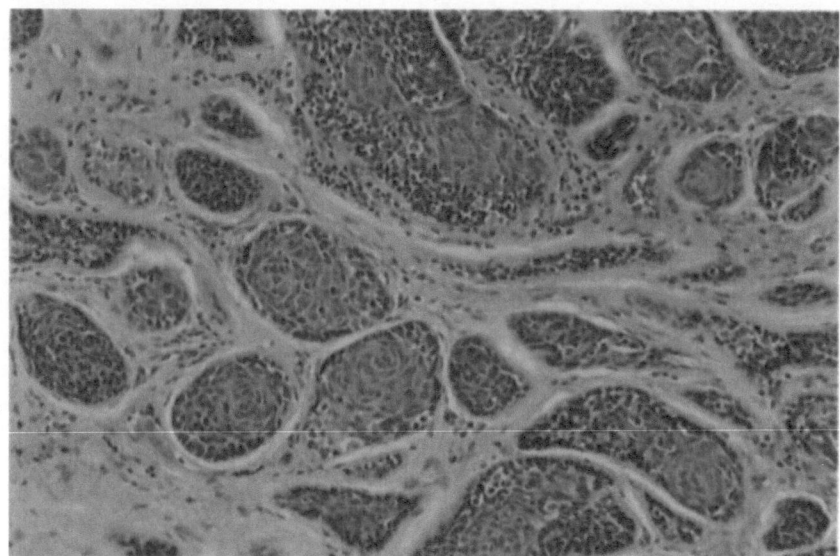

Fig. 65. *Basal cell adenocarcinoma*
Solid type with small dark cells and large pale cells

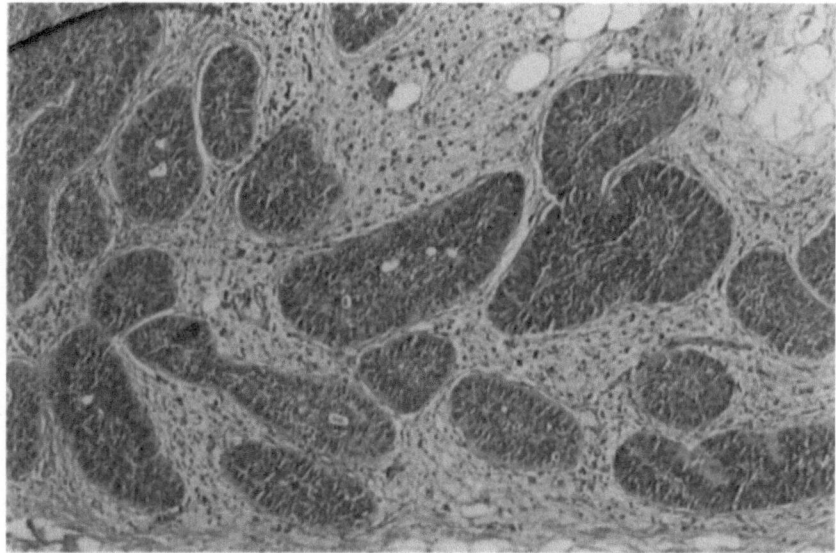

Fig. 66. *Basal cell adenocarcinoma*
Trabecular type with thin hyaline material on the outside and distinct demarcation from the fibrous connective tissue stroma

84

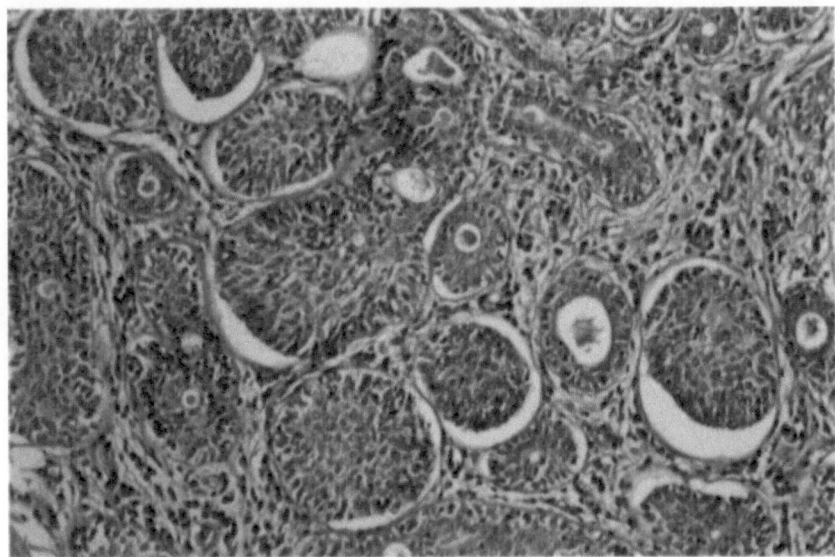

Fig. 67. *Basal cell adenocarcinoma*
Mixed trabecular and tubular type

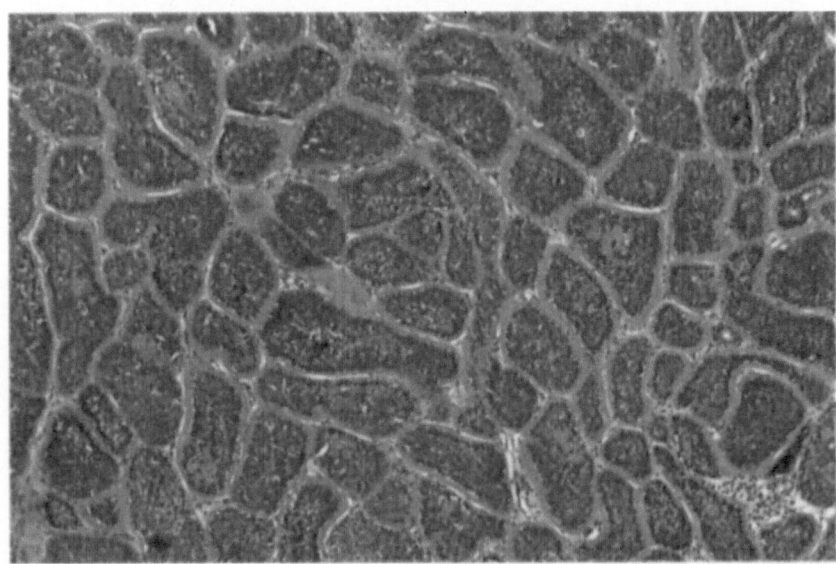

Fig. 68. *Basal cell adenocarcinoma*
Membranous type with surrounding hyaline lamina

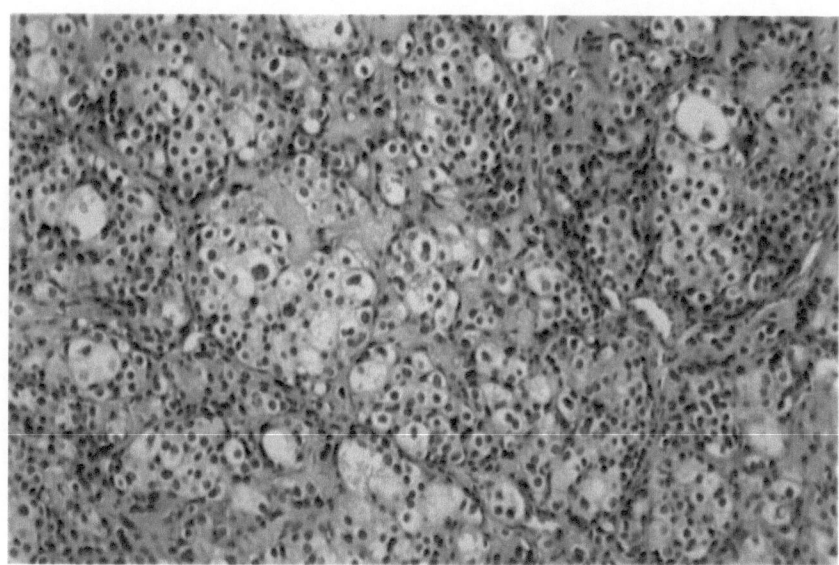

Fig. 69. *Sebaceous carcinoma*
Nests of sebaceous cells in lobular arrangement

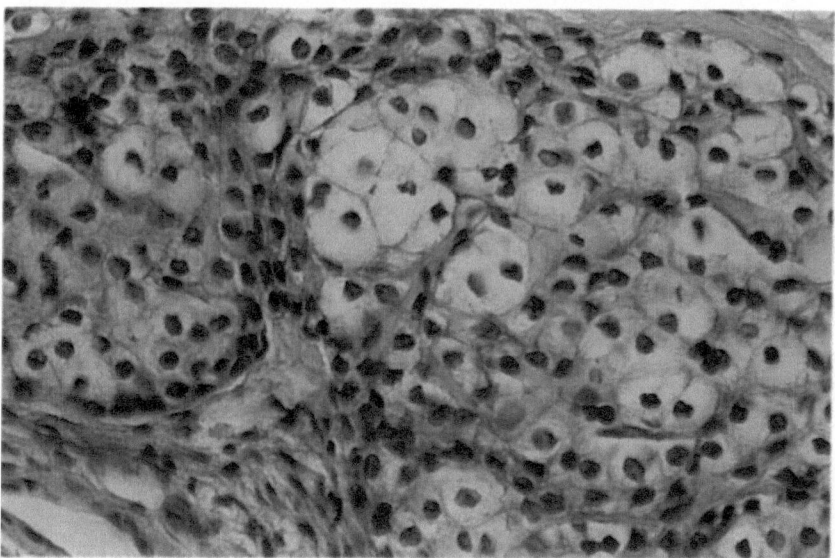

Fig. 70. *Sebaceous carcinoma*
Sebaceous cells with distinct cellular membrane and vacuolated cytoplasm

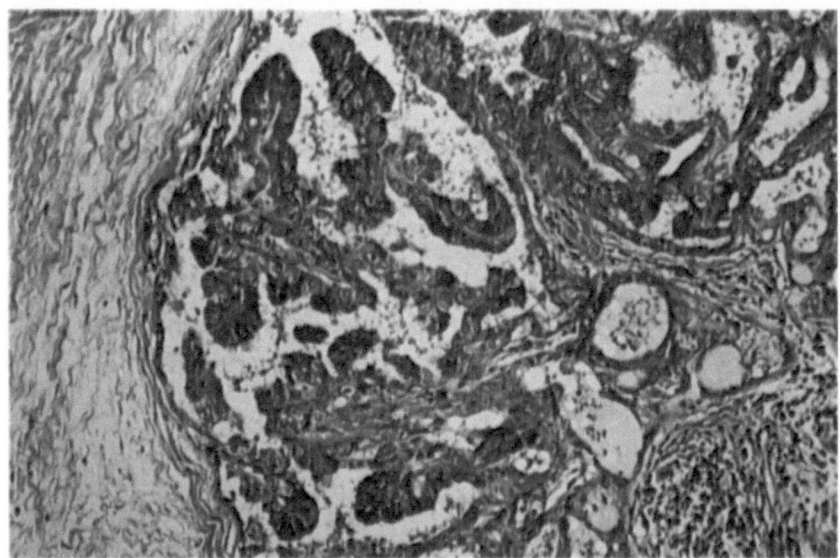

Fig. 71. *Papillary cystadenocarcinoma*
Cysts with papillary endocystic projections

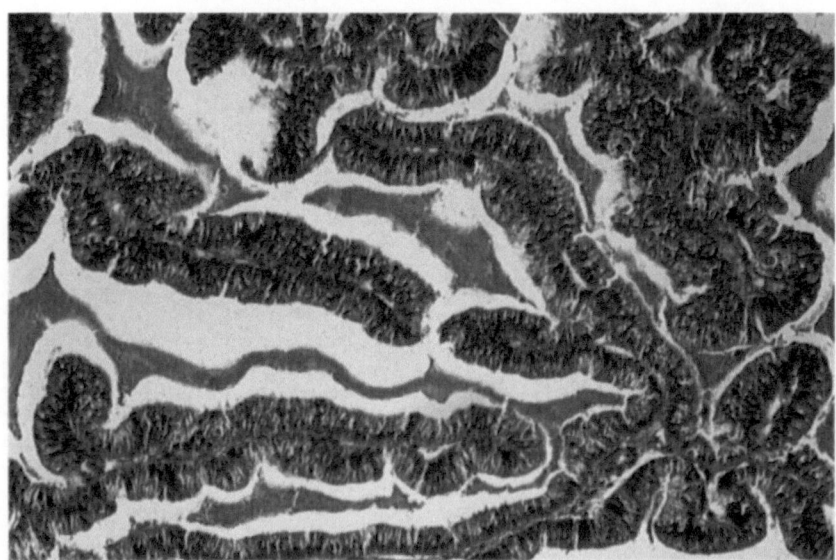

Fig. 72. *Papillary cystadenocarcinoma*
Papillary projections with narrow fibrous cores

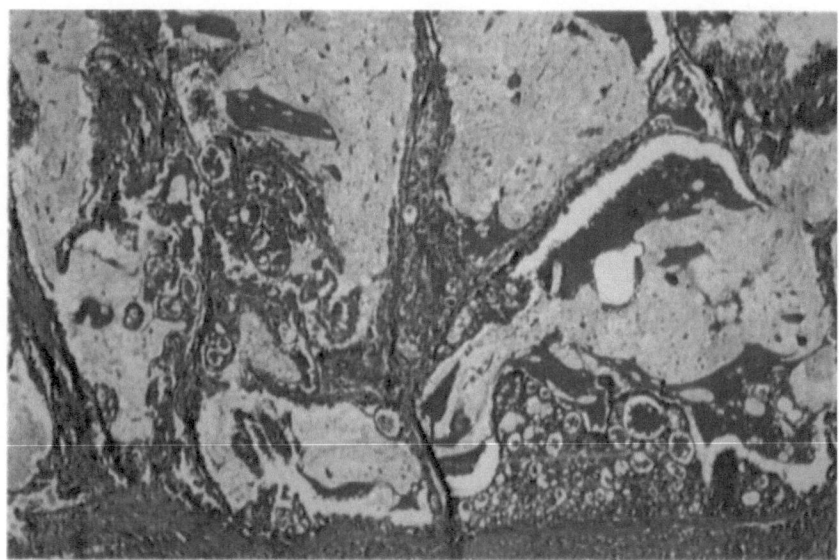

Fig. 73. *Mucinous adenocarcinoma*
Multiple cystic spaces with mucus production

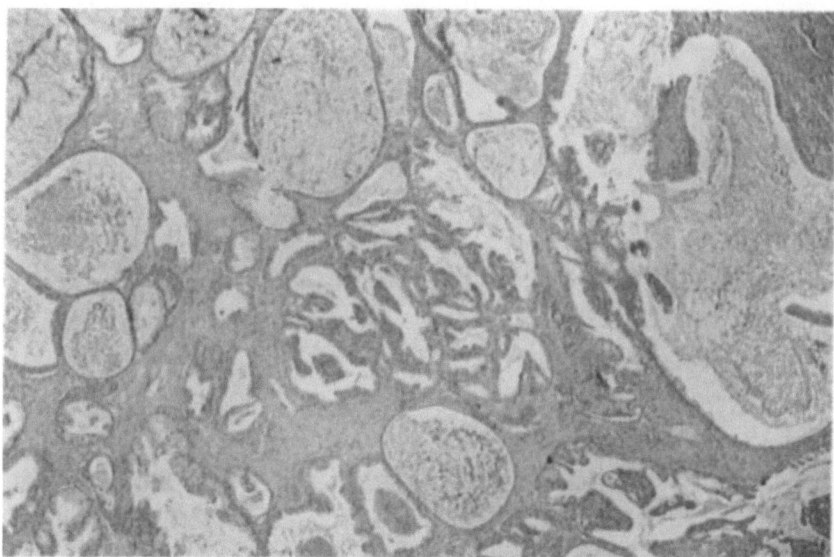

Fig. 74. *Mucinous adenocarcinoma*
Mucus in the cystic spaces. Astra blue

88

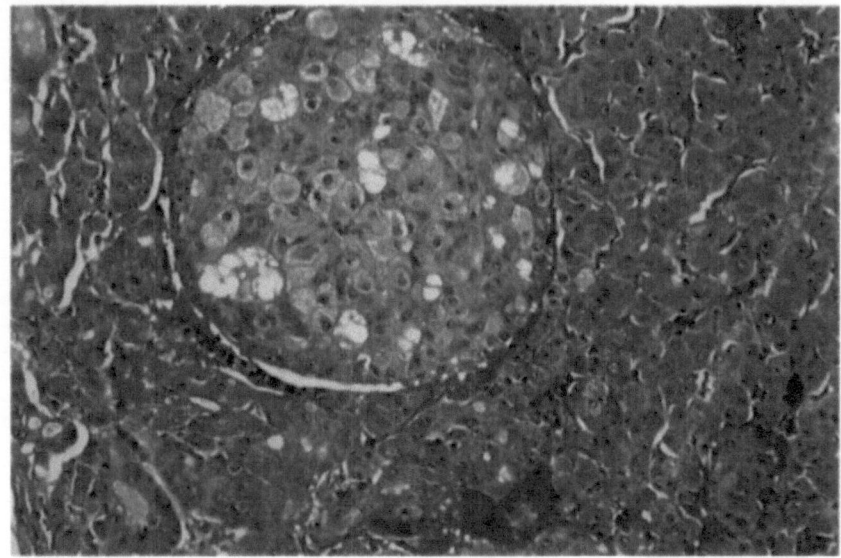

Fig. 75. *Oncocytic carcinoma*
Compact nests of eosinophilic cells

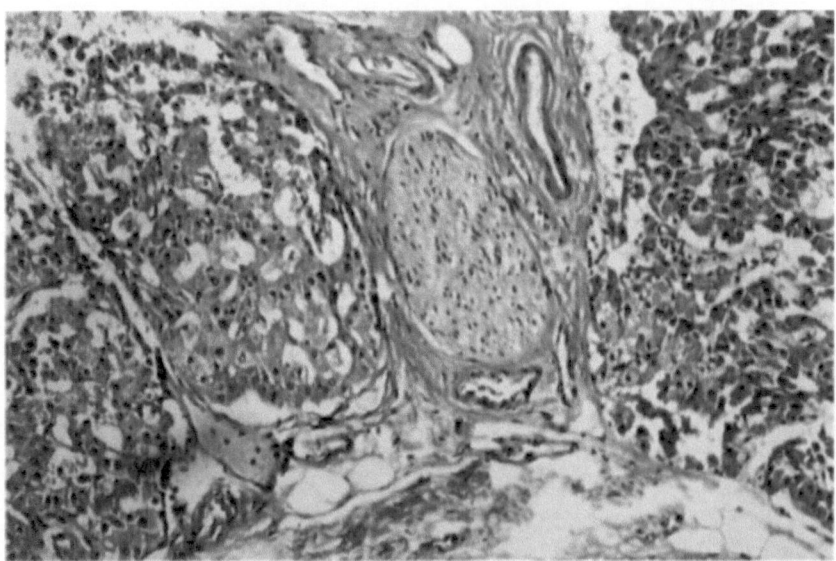

Fig. 76. *Oncocytic carcinoma*
Infiltrating growth near nerve

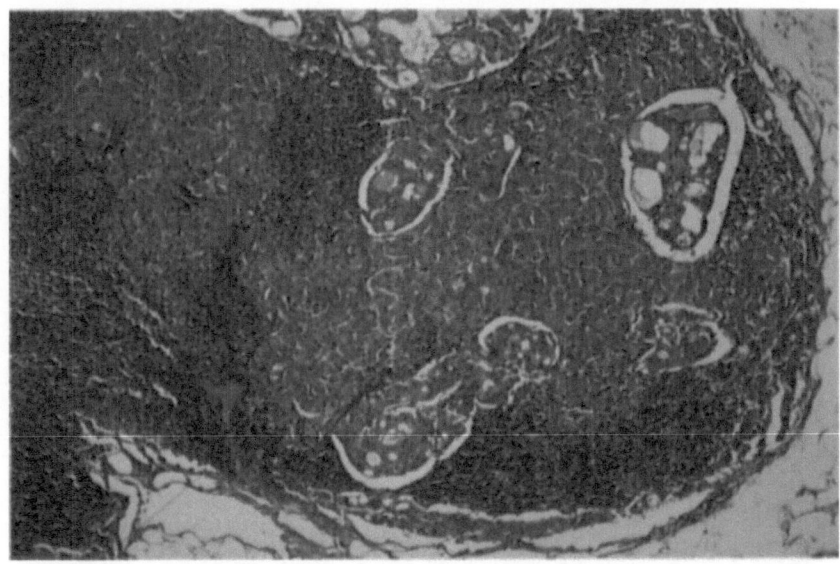

Fig. 77. *Oncocytic carcinoma*
Lymph node metastasis

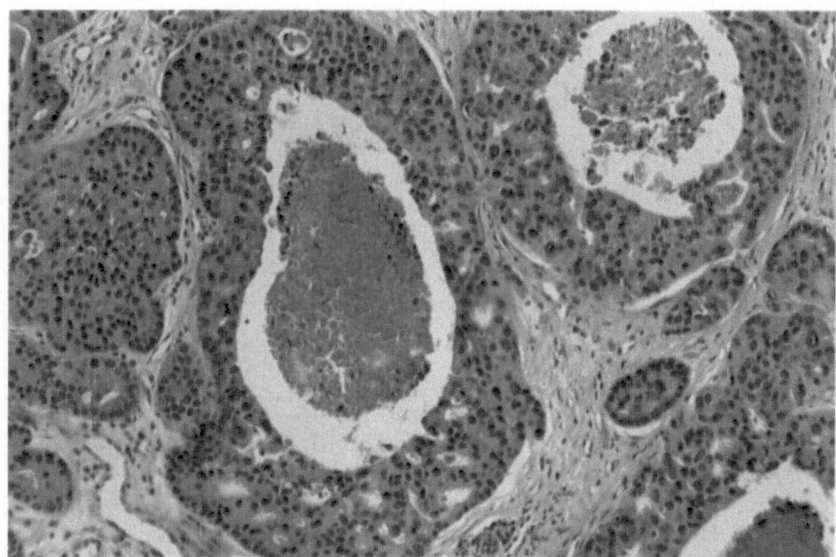

Fig. 78. *Salivary duct carcinoma*
Cribriform pattern with central necrosis

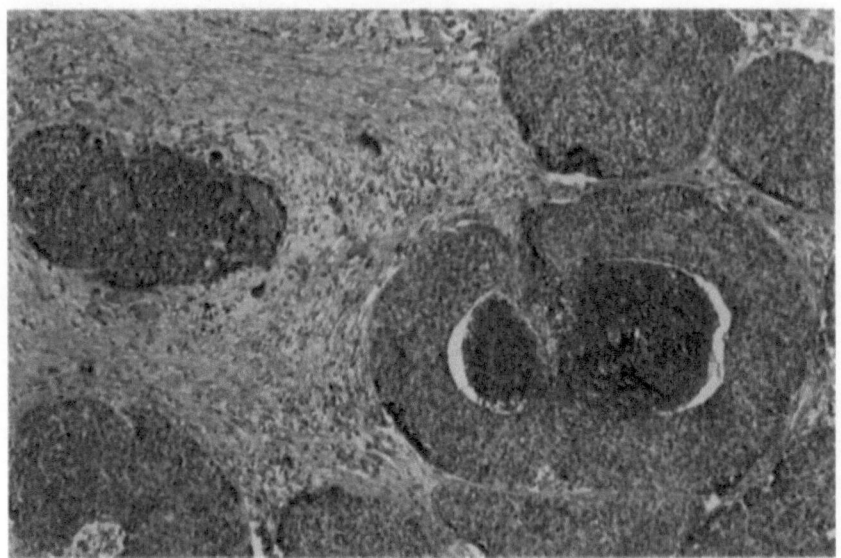

Fig. 79. *Salivary duct carcinoma*
Solid pattern with central necrosis

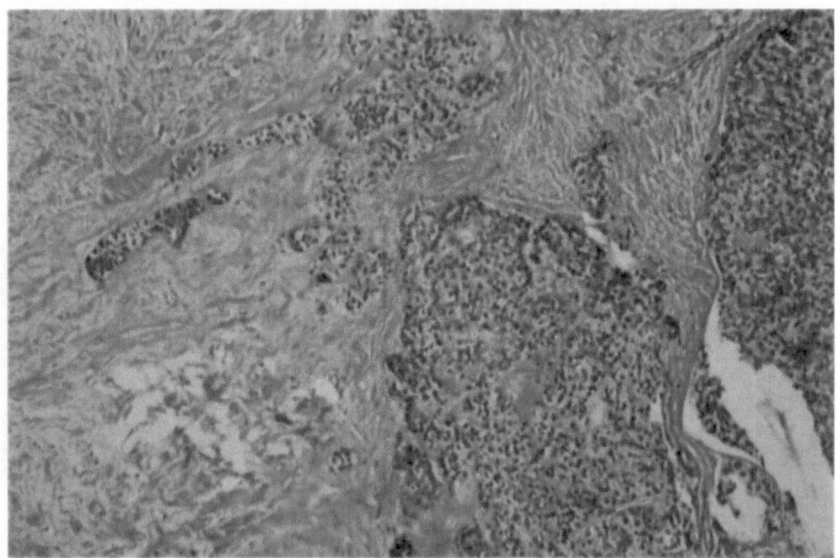

Fig. 80. *Malignant myoepithelioma*
Infiltrating growth with a conspicuous stroma

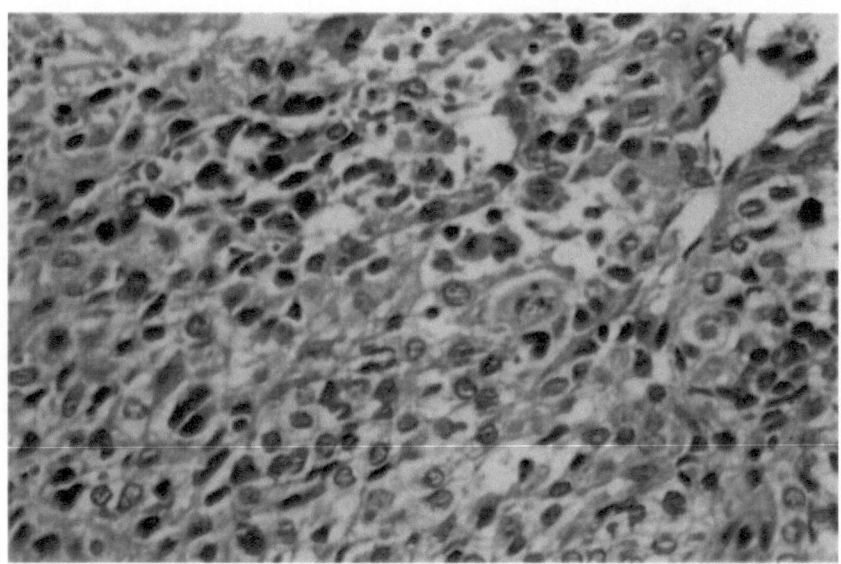

Fig. 81. *Malignant myoepithelioma*
Atypical myoepithelial cells with prominent mitotic activity

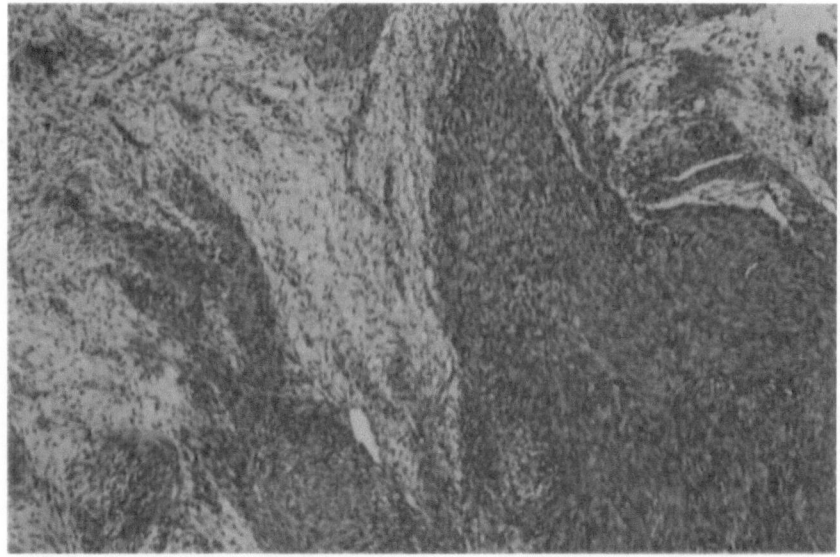

Fig. 82. *Malignant myoepithelioma*
Sarcoma-like structure with spindle-shaped cells and aggressive growth

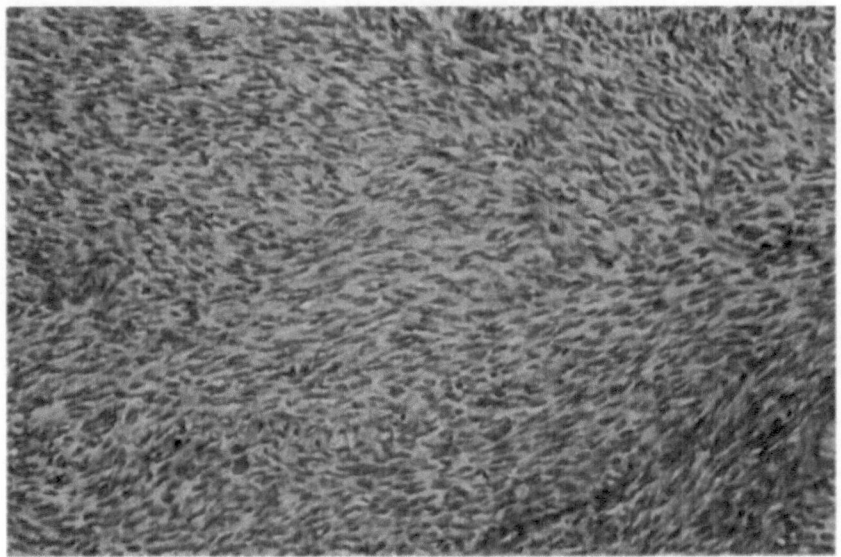

Fig. 83. *Malignant myoepithelioma*
Spindle-shaped cell type

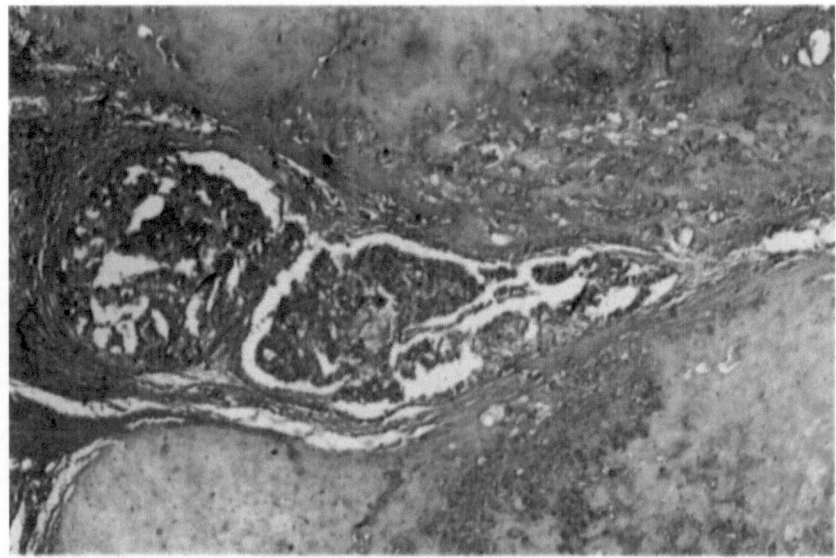

Fig. 84. *Carcinoma in pleomorphic adenoma*
Carcinomatous area *(left side)* in a pleomorphic adenoma

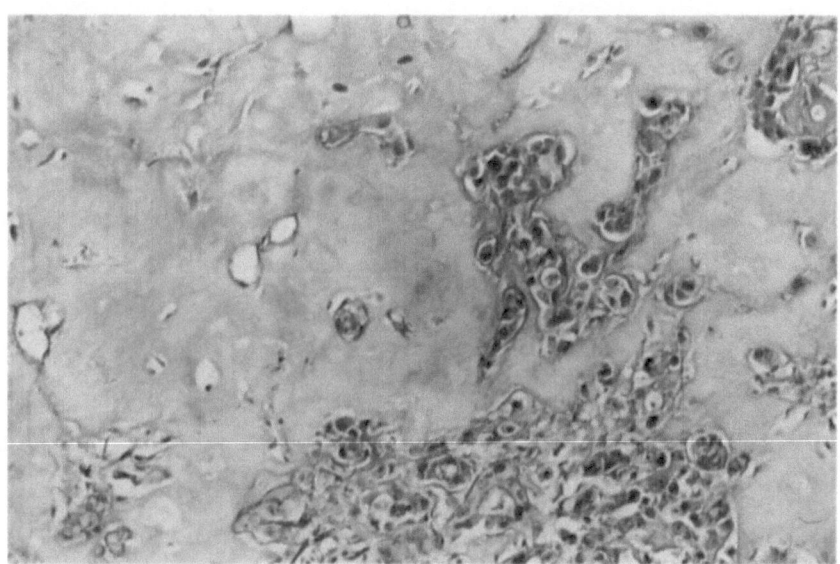

Fig. 85. *Carcinoma in pleomorphic adenoma*
Hyalinization of the stroma with nests of carcinoma. Periodic acid-Schiff

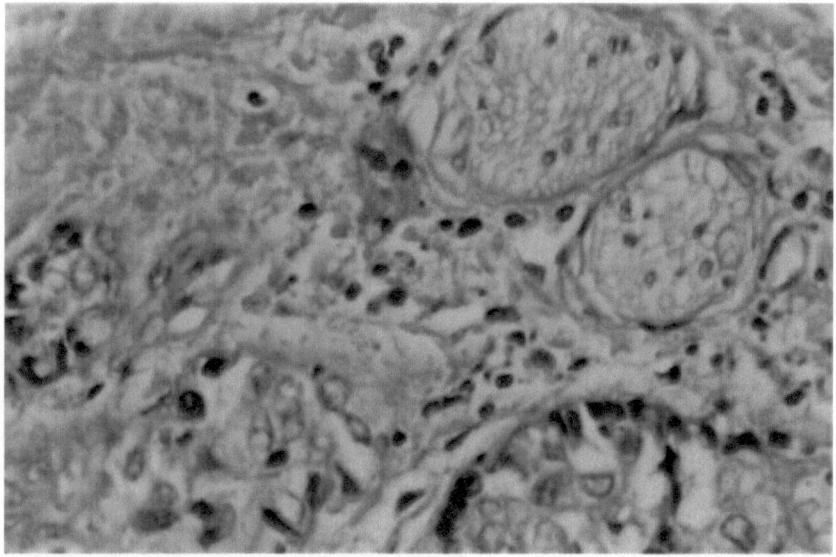

Fig. 86. *Carcinoma in pleomorphic adenoma*
Infiltrating growth with perineural invasion

94

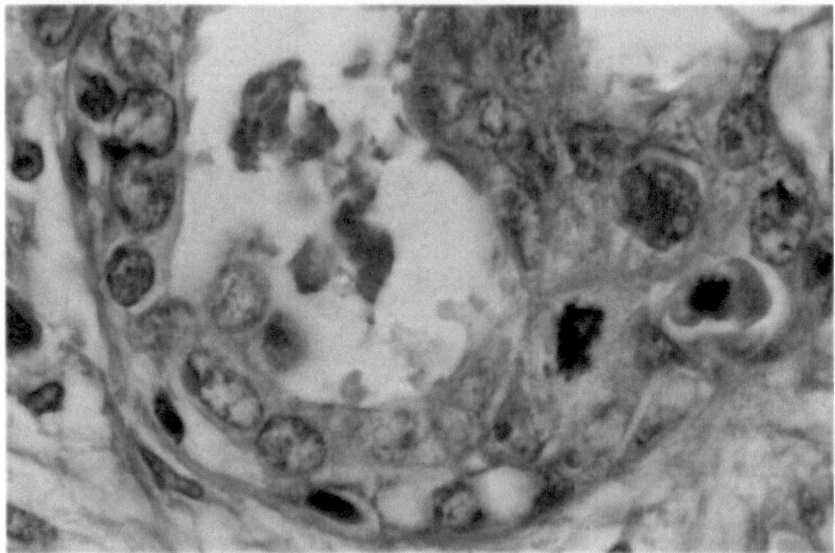

Fig. 87. *Carcinoma in pleomorphic adenoma*
Cellular anaplasia and abnormal mitoses

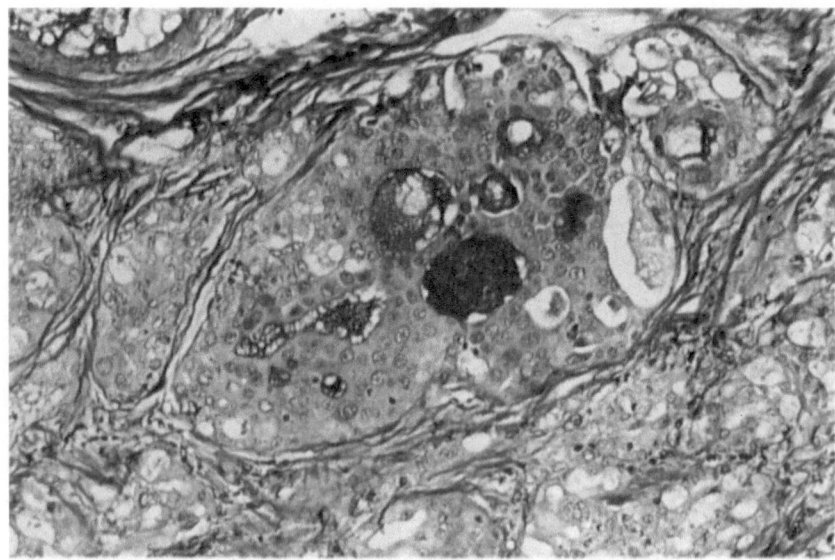

Fig. 88. *Carcinoma in pleomorphic adenoma*
Mucoepidermoid carcinoma in a pleomorphic adenoma. Periodic acid-Schiff

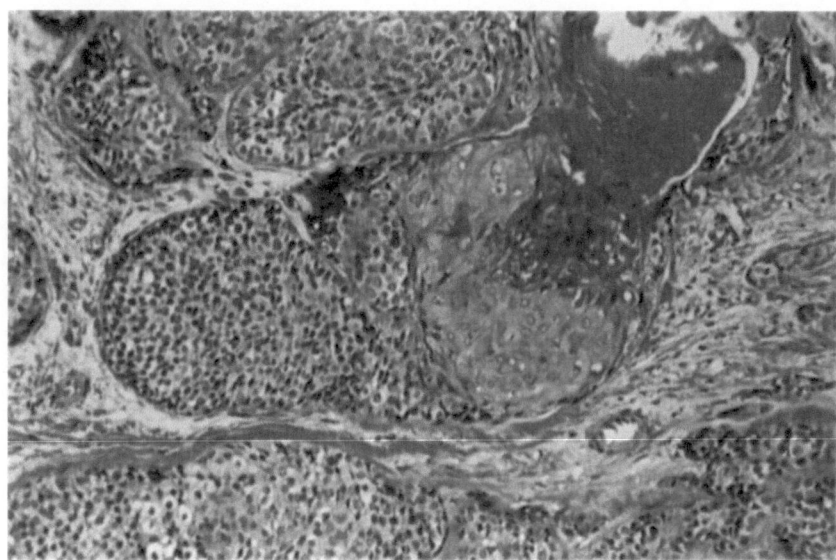

Fig. 89. *Carcinoma in pleomorphic adenoma*
Undifferentiated growth with squamous focus

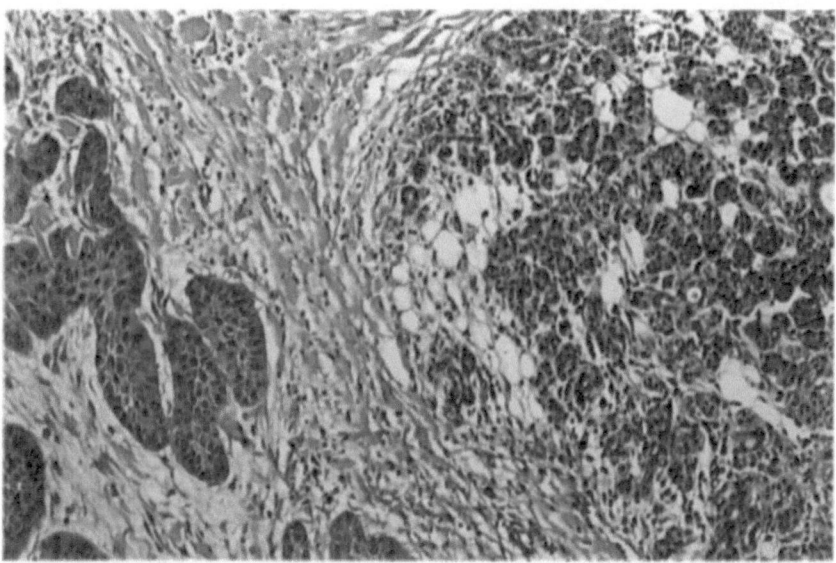

Fig. 90. *Squamous cell carcinoma*
Non-keratinized infiltrating cell nests

96

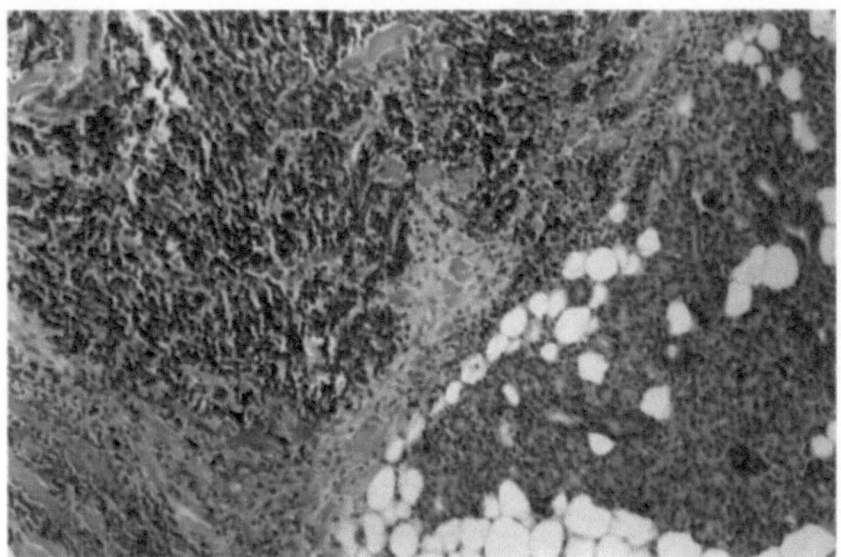

Fig.91. *Small cell carcinoma*

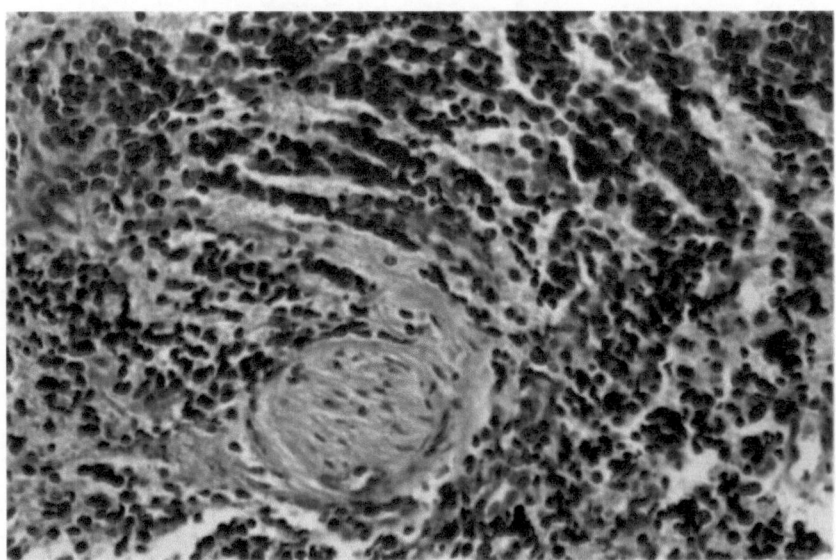

Fig.92. *Small cell carcinoma*
Perineural infiltration

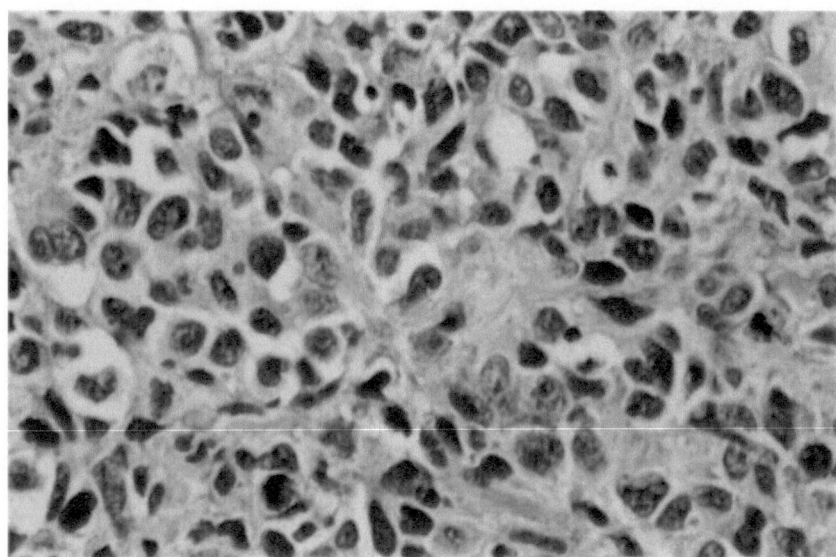

Fig. 93. *Undifferentiated carcinoma*
Mixture of large and spindle cells

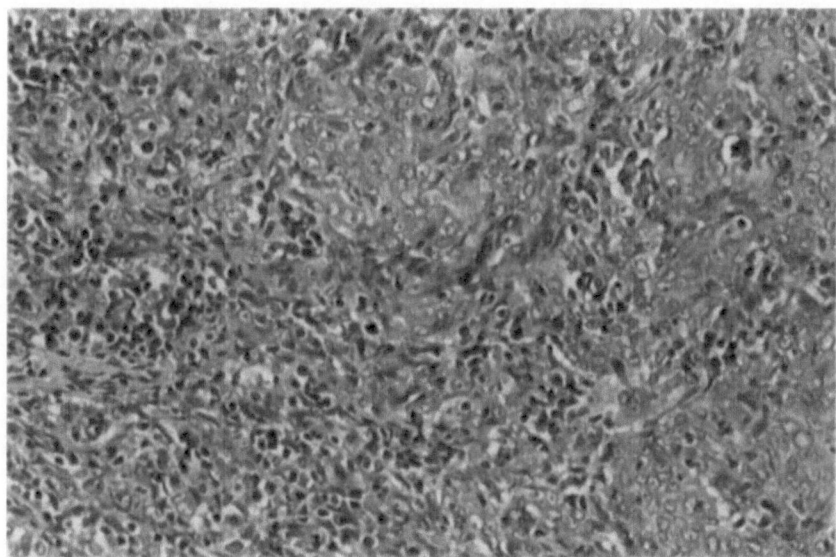

Fig. 94. *Undifferentiated carcinoma with lymphoid stroma*
Clumps of large cells with vesicular nuclei, admixed with abundant lymphocytes

98

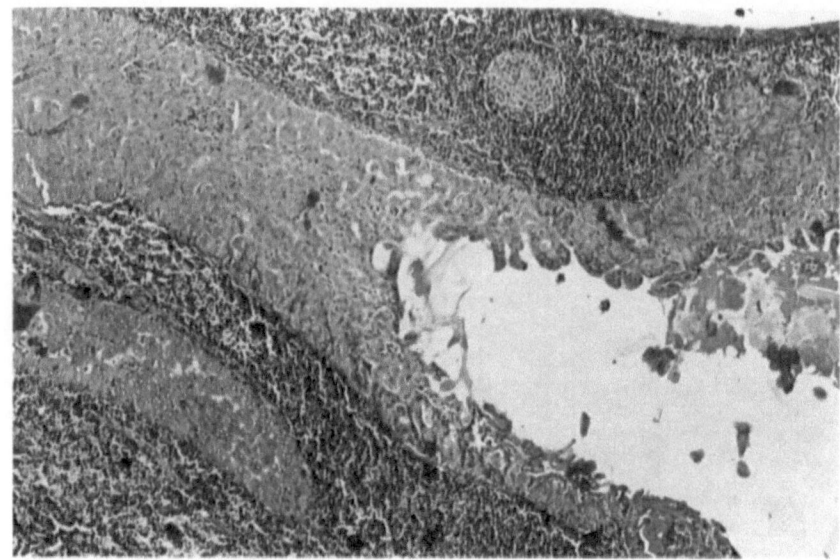

Fig. 95. *Carcinoma in Warthin tumour*
Carcinomatous endocystic papillary proliferation (analogous to acinic cell carcinoma)

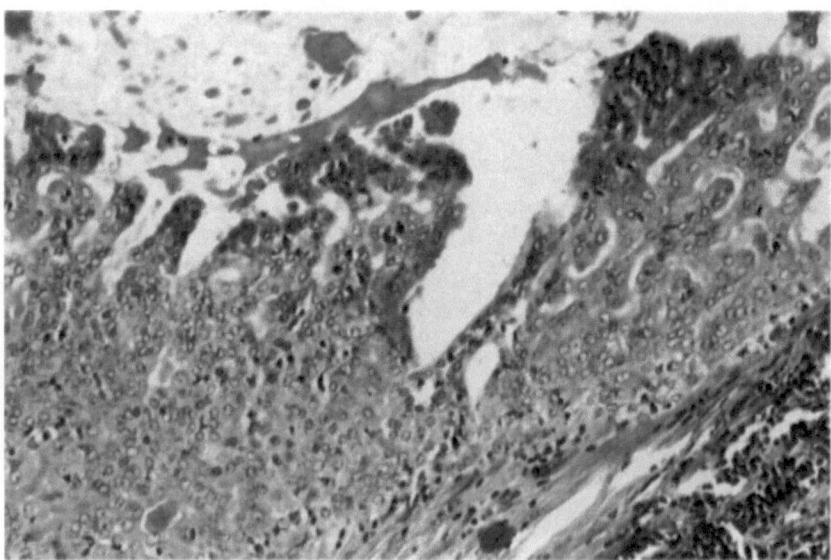

Fig. 96. *Carcinoma in Warthin tumour*
Atypical papillary projections. Same case as Fig. 95

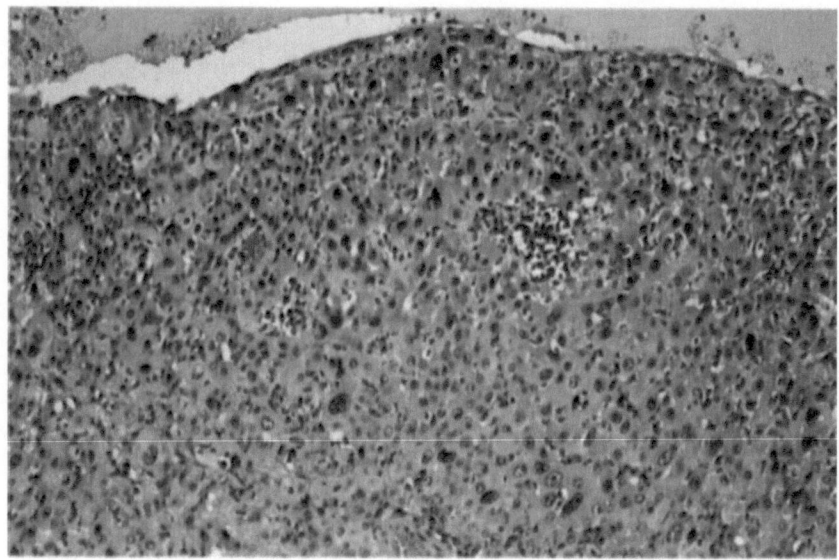

Fig. 97. *Carcinoma in Warthin tumour*
Solid nests of atypical squamous cells

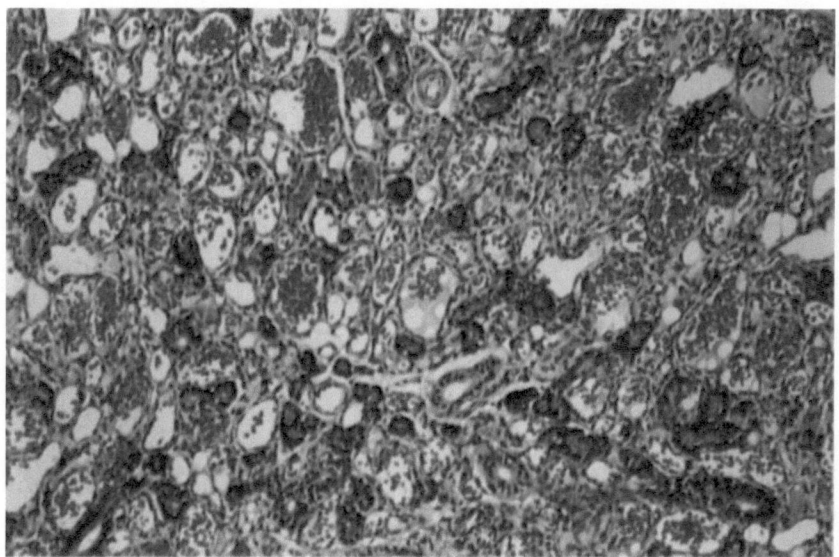

Fig. 98. *Haemangioma*
Separation and reduction of the parotid tissue by angiomatous proliferation

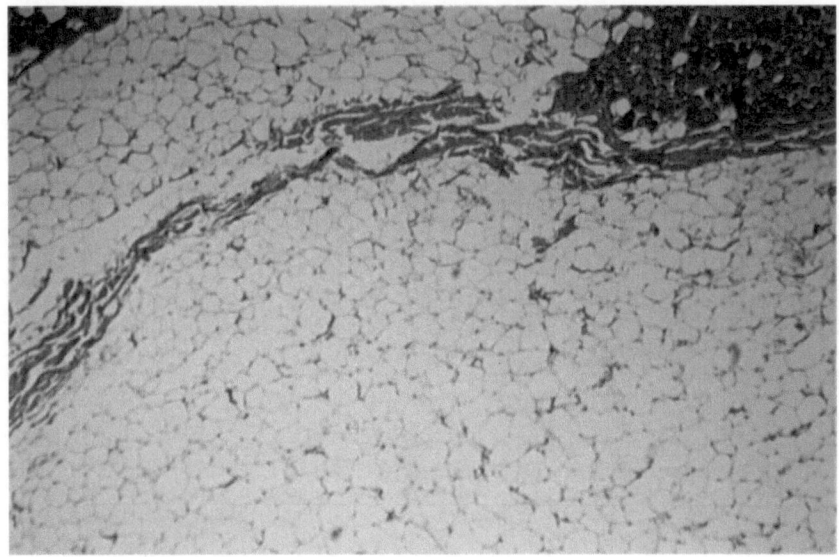

Fig. 99. *Lipoma*
Replacement of the parotid gland parenchyma by fatty tissue

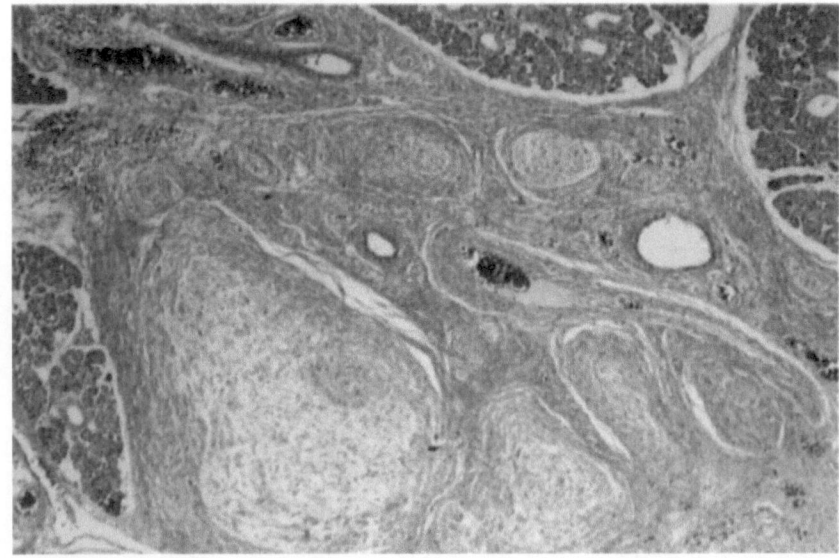

Fig. 100. *Neurofibromatosis*
Multifocal nodular neural proliferations. Masson-Goldner

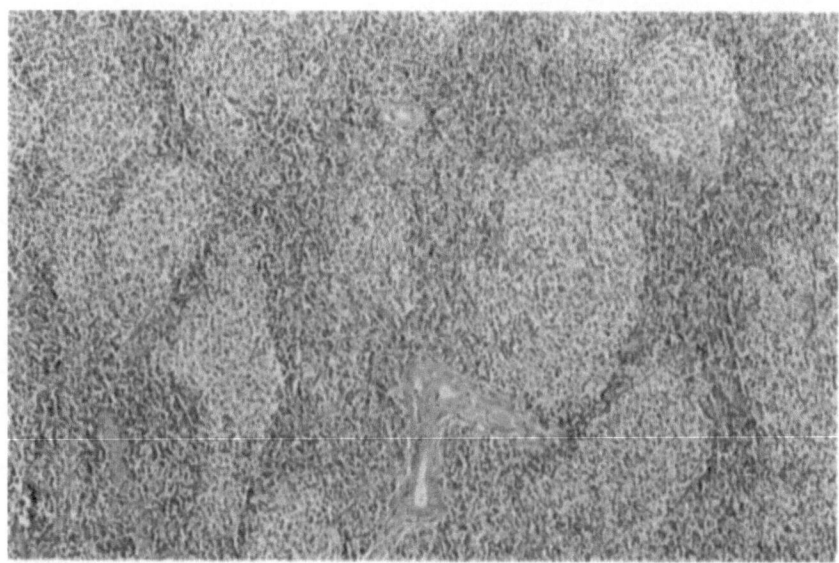

Fig. 101. *Malignant lymphoma (low-grade follicular centrocytic-centroblastic type)*
Duct remnants among the lymphoid infiltrate

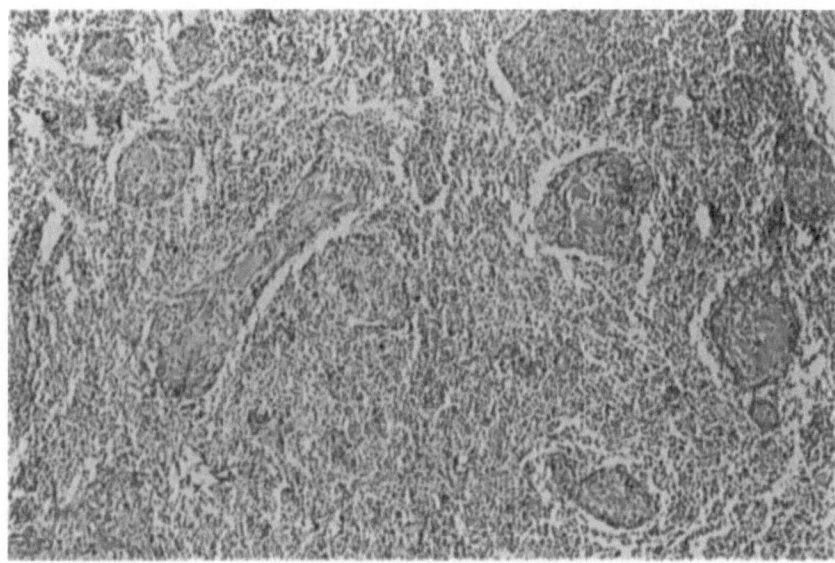

Fig. 102. *Malignant lymphoma (high-grade immunoblastic type)*
Associated with chronic immunosialadenitis (remnants of epimyoepithelial cell islands)

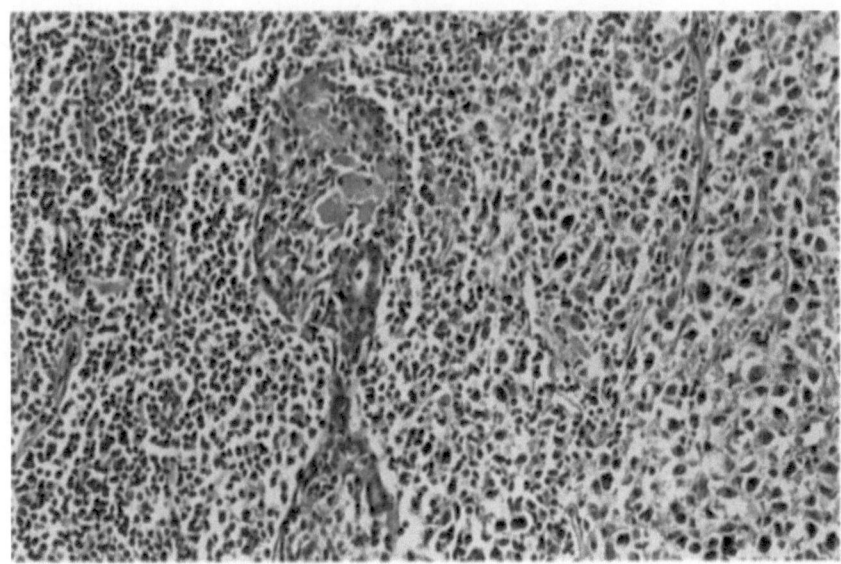

Fig. 103. *Malignant lymphoma (immunoblastic type)*
Same case as Fig. 102, higher magnification

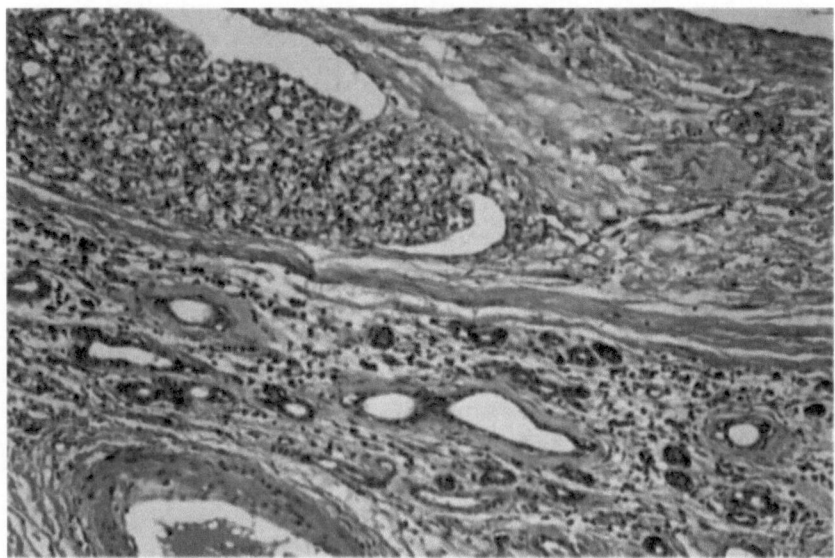

Fig. 104. *Metastasis* of a renal cell carcinoma
Clear cell tumour nests in a blood vessel of the parotid gland

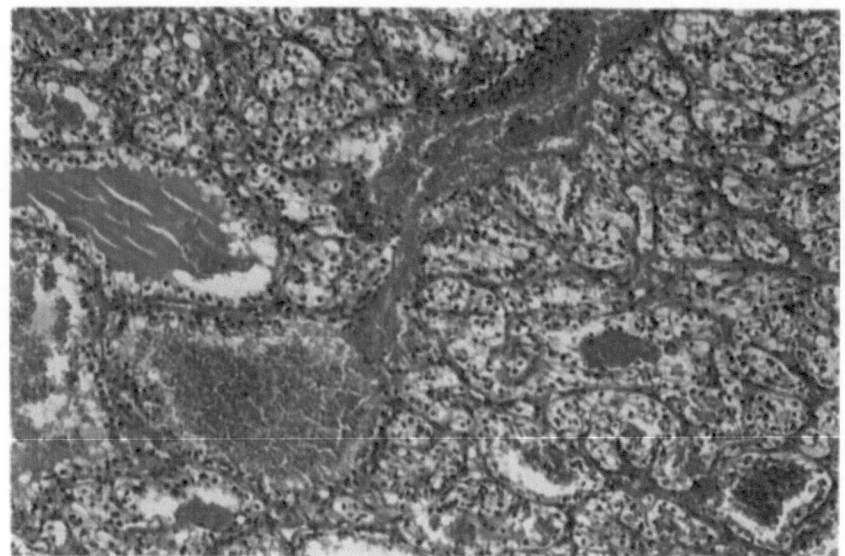

Fig. 105. *Metastasis* of a renal cell carcinoma
High vascularization of the tumour stroma. Same case as Fig. 104

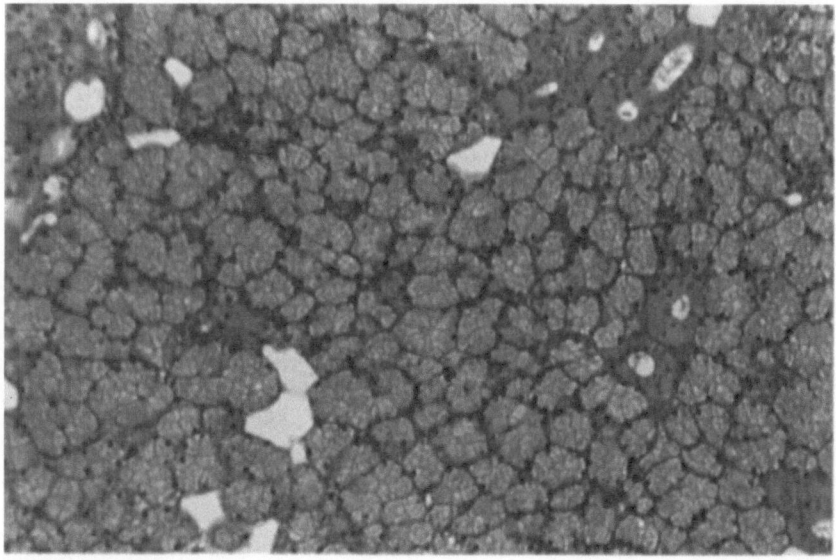

Fig. 106. *Sialadenosis*
Swollen acini of the parotid gland with slight compression of the ducts. No sign
of inflammation

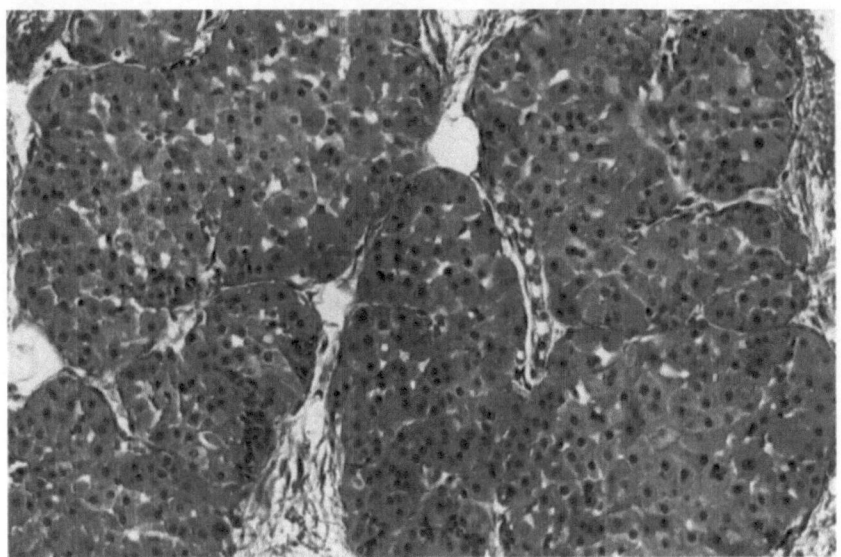

Fig. 107. *Diffuse oncocytosis*
Complete oncocytic metaplasia of the parotid gland lobules

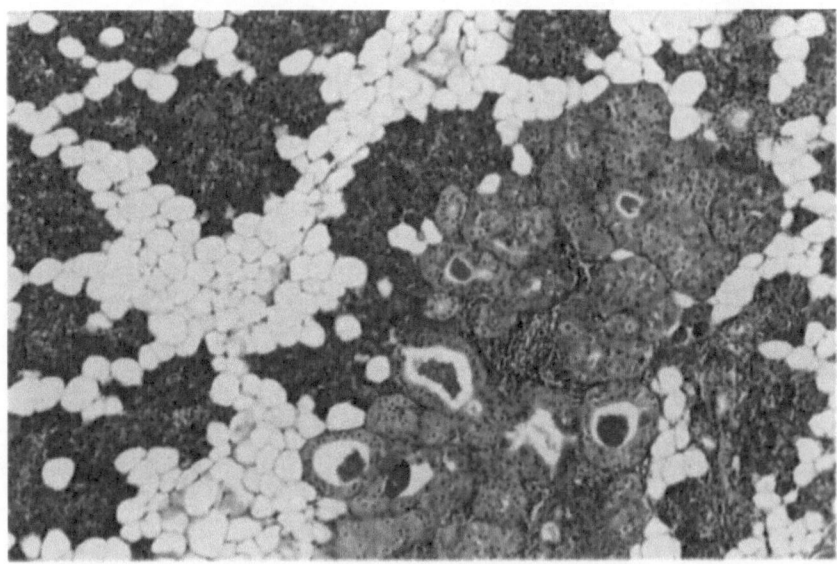

Fig. 108. *Multifocal oncocytic adenomatous hyperplasia*
Parotid gland lobule with micronodular hyperplasia of oncocytic foci

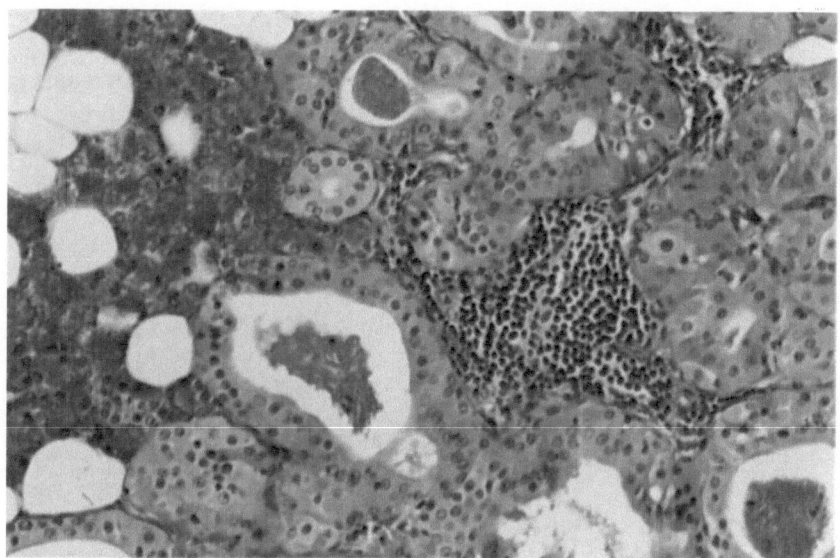

Fig. 109. *Multifocal oncocytic adenomatous hyperplasia*
Remnants of parotid gland acini *(left side)*. Same case as Fig. 108

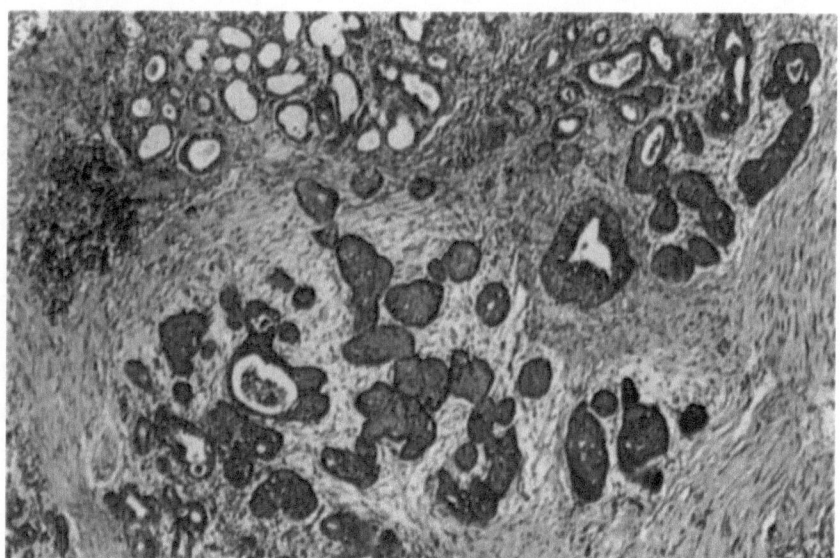

Fig. 110. *Necrotizing sialometaplasia*
Lobular arrangement with squamous metaplasia of the duct system. Masson-Goldner

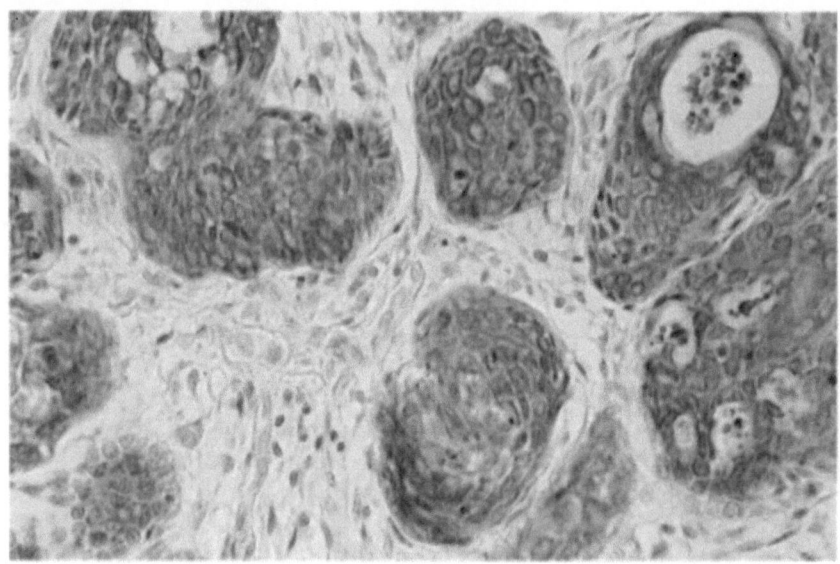

Fig. 111. *Necrotizing sialometaplasia*
Positive cytokeratin reaction of the metaplastic areas. Immunocytochemical
peroxidase-antiperoxidase method

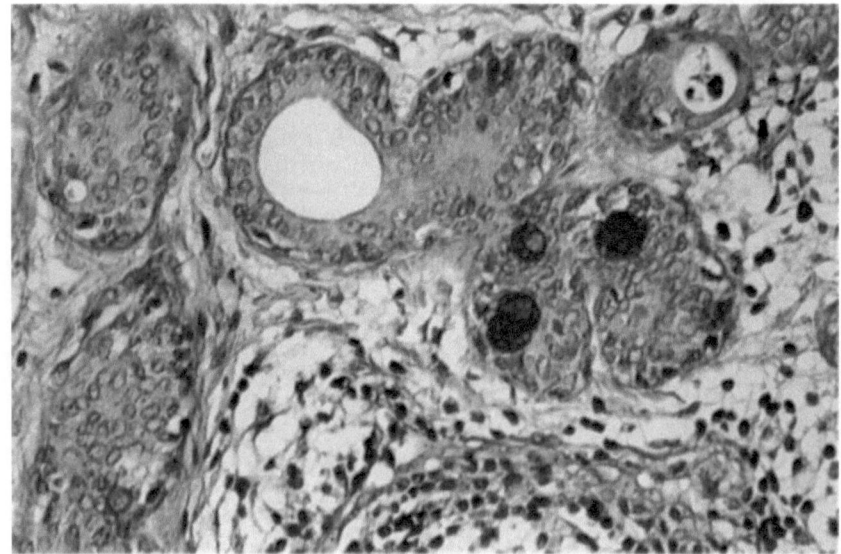

Fig. 112. *Necrotizing sialometaplasia*
Goblet cells within the squamous cell metaplasia. Periodic acid-Schiff

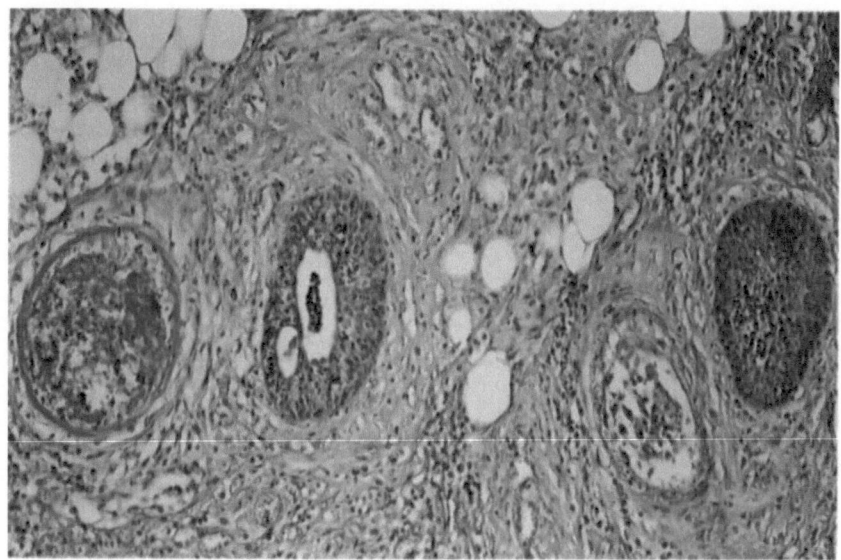

Fig. 113. *Necrotizing sialometaplasia*
Vascular changes (thrombosis) around salivary gland infarct

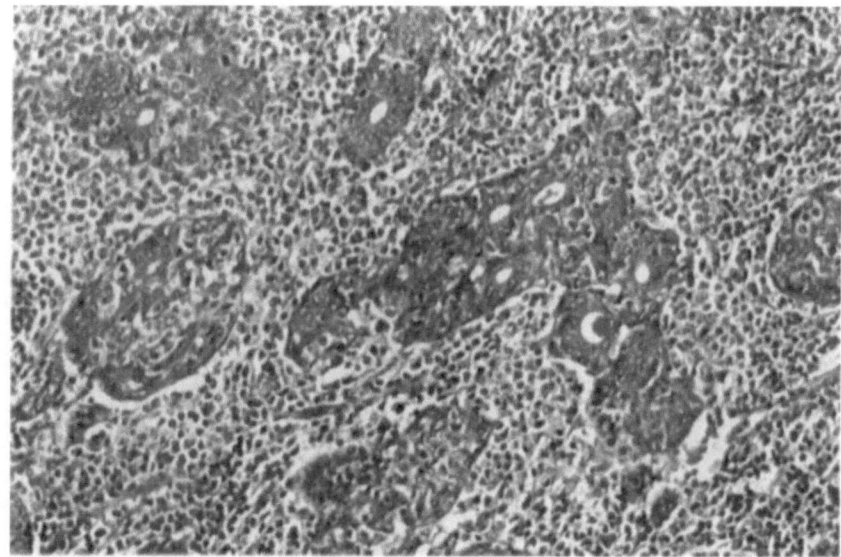

Fig. 114. *Benign lymphoepithelial lesion*
Diffuse interstitial lymphocytic infiltration of the parotid gland with inclusion of
epimyoepithelial cell islands

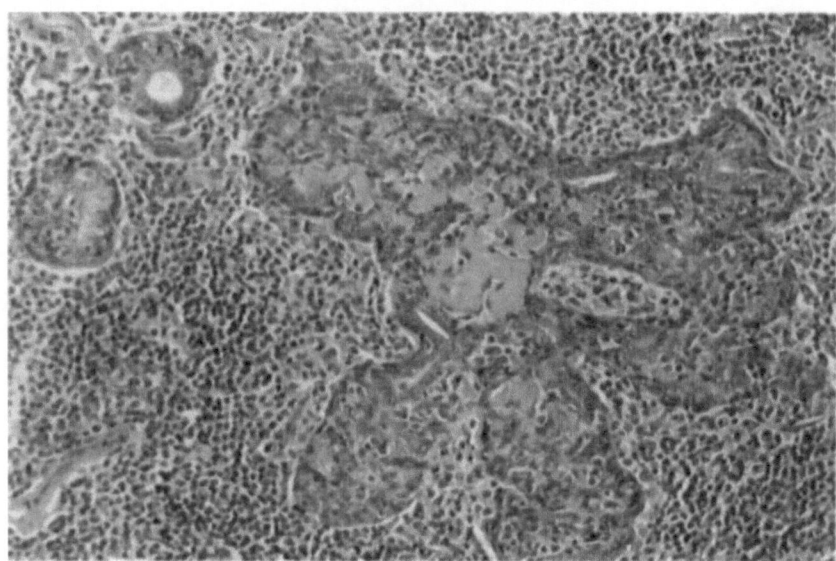

Fig. 115. *Benign lymphoepithelial lesion*
Hyaline tranformation of an epimyoepithelial cell island

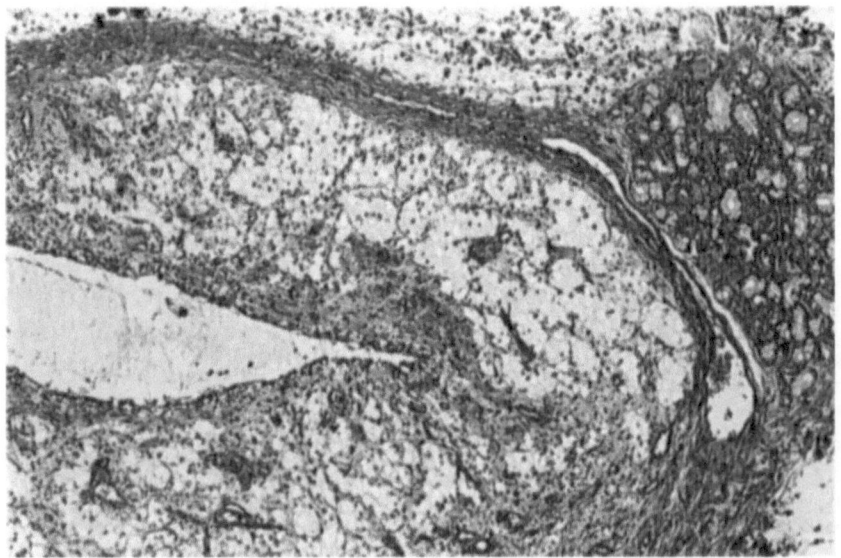

Fig. 116. *Extravasated cyst (mucocele)*
Mucus-filled pseudocyst with a connective tissue capsule

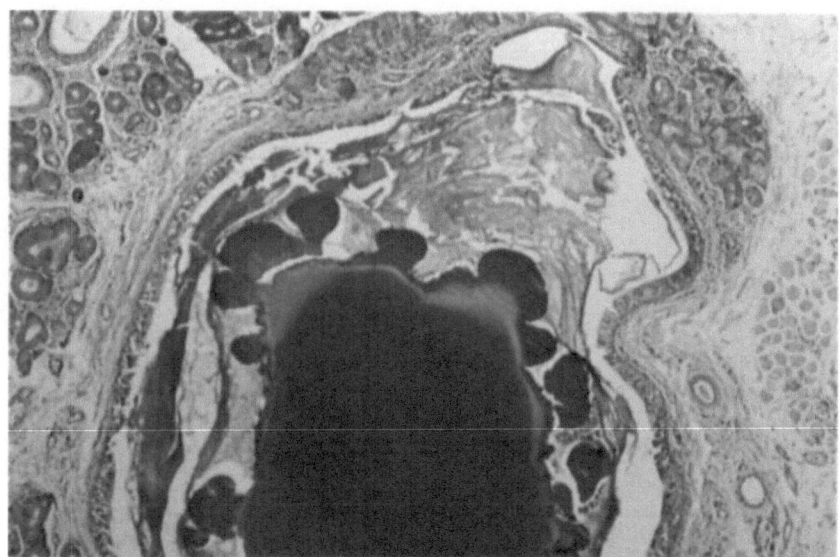

Fig. 117. *Retention cyst*
Epithelial lining of the cyst with viscous mucus retention. Periodic acid-Schiff

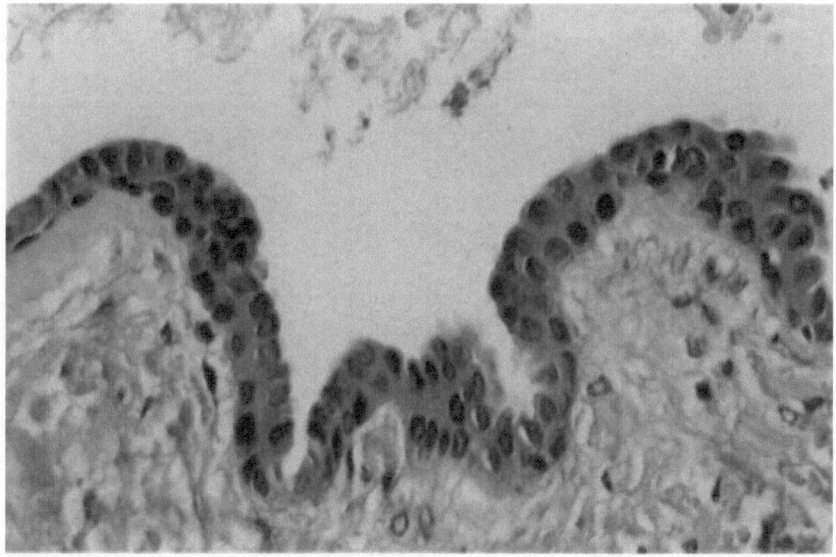

Fig. 118. *Salivary duct cyst*
Lining by a double layer of duct epithelium

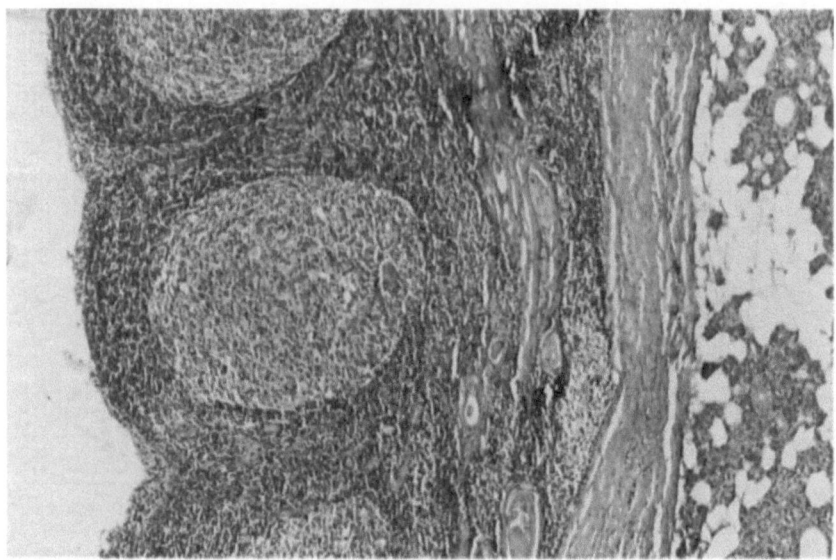

Fig. 119. *Lymphoepithelial cyst*
Lining by multilayered epithelium and a lymphoid stroma with lymph follicles

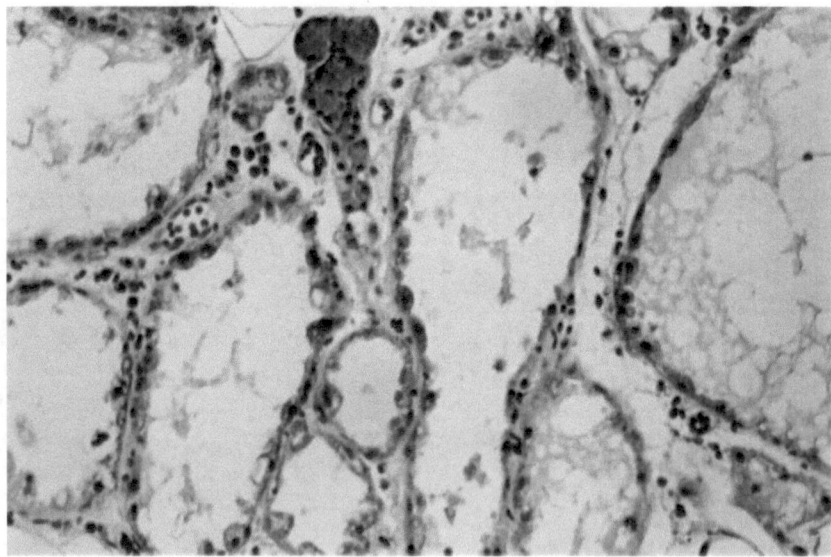

Fig. 120. *Dysgenetic polycystic disease*
Multiple duct-like cysts and remnants of parotid gland acini. Masson-Goldner

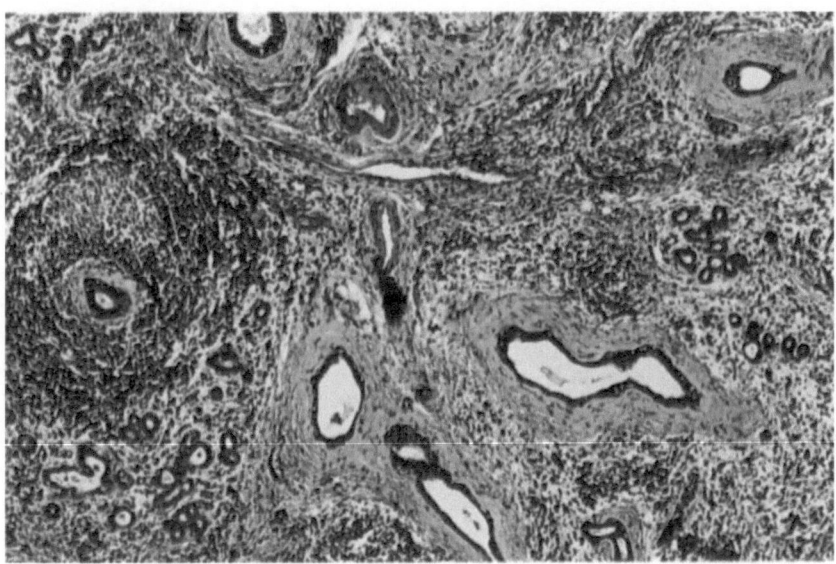

Fig. 121. *Chronic sclerosing sialadenitis of submandibular gland (Küttner tumour)*
Periductal sclerosis, lymphocytic infiltration and reduction of the secretory gland parenchyma

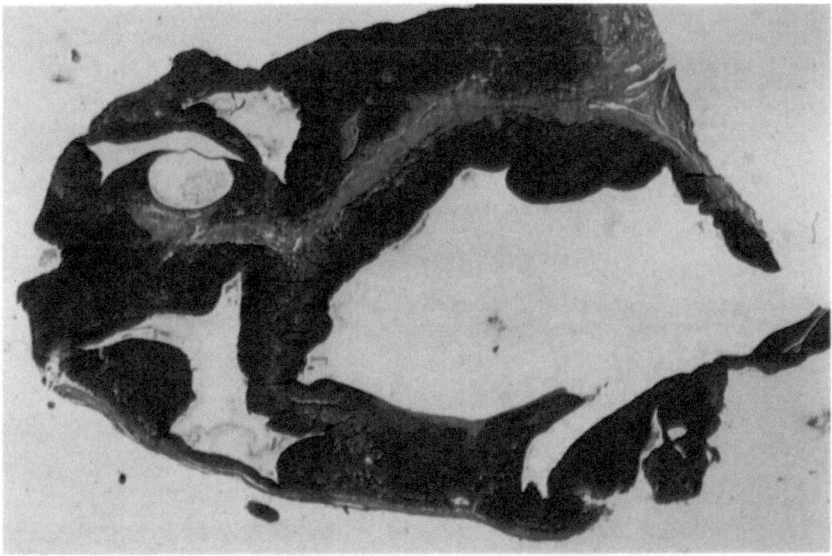

Fig. 122. *Cystic lymphoid hyperplasia in AIDS*
Gross epithelial cysts within lymph nodes

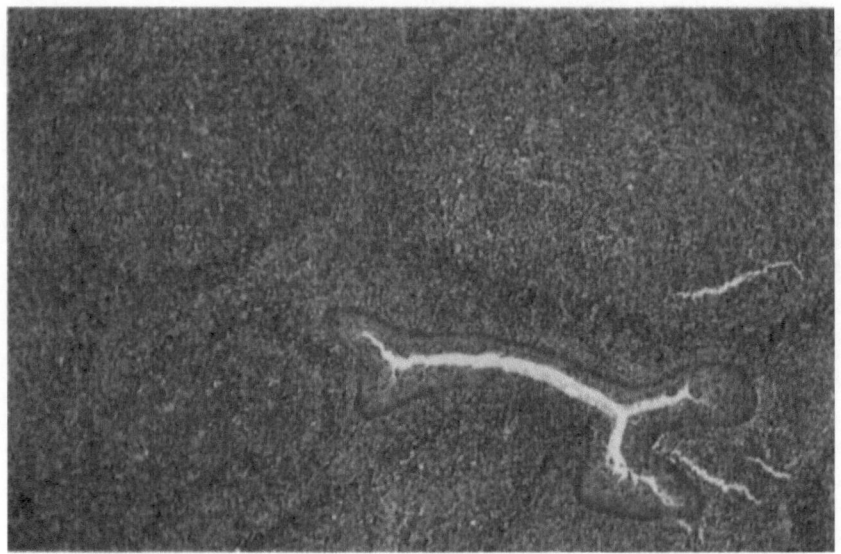

Fig. 123. *Cystic lymphoid hyperplasia in AIDS*
Cyst lined by invaginating squamous epithelium and surrounded by reactive
lymphoid hyperplasia

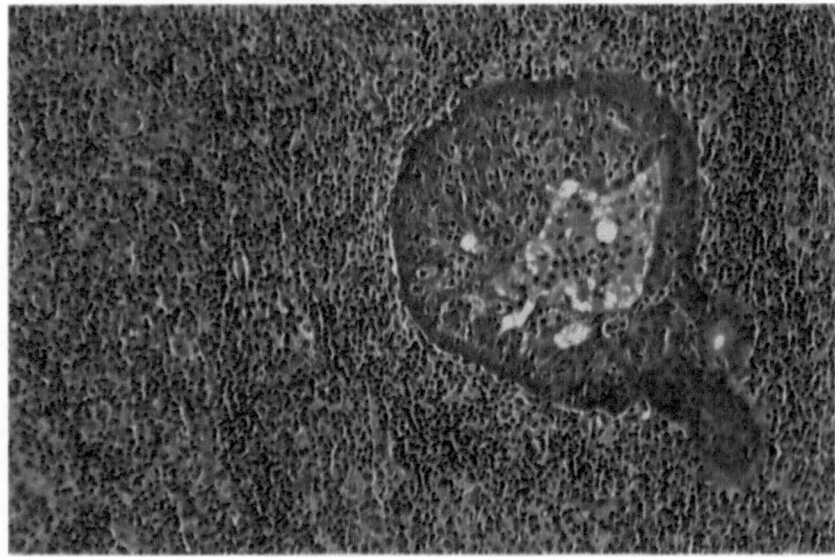

Fig. 124. *Cystic lymphoid hyperplasia in AIDS*
Inclusion of an epimyoepithelial cell island

WHO International Histological Classification of Tumours
Seifert et al.: Histological Typing of Salivary Gland Tumours,
2nd edn.

---

35 mm Colour Transparencies

A set of 124 colour slides (35 mm), corresponding to the photomicrographs in this book, is available from the American Registry of Pathology. To order these *slides,* send the following information to:

American Registry of Pathology
14th Street and Alaska Ave. NW
Washington, DC 20306 USA

Please send me:

_____ set(s) of 35 mm slides of Histological Typing of Salivary Gland Tumours at $ 70 per set.
For Air Mail outside of North America add $ 10.00.

Total cost: $ _____ .00

Name _____

Address _____

_____

_____

Date _____ Signature _____

☐ I enclose a check/money order in US$ payable to the ARP.
☐ Please charge my credit card:
    ☐ VISA
    ☐ MasterCard

Card number _____

Expiration date _____

Name as it appears on credit card _____

Prices are subject to change without notice.

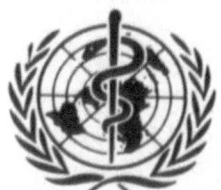

World Health Organization
International Histological
Classification of Tumours

Histological Typing of . . .

C. Hedinger

Histological Typing of

Thyroid Tumours

In Collaboration with E. D. Williams and L. H. Sobin

2nd ed. 1988. XII, 67 pp. 92 figs. Softcover. ISBN 3-540-19244-1

J. R. Jass, L. H. Sobin

Histological Typing of

Intestinal Tumours

2nd ed. 1989. XII, 127 pp. 136 figs. Softcover. ISBN 3-540-50711-6

H. Watanabe, J. R. Jass, L. H. Sobin

Histological Typing of

Oesophageal and Gastric Tumours

2nd ed. 1990. XII, 109 pp. 120 figs. 4 tabs. Softcover. ISBN 3-540-51629-8

J. Albores-Saavedra, D. E. Henson, L. H. Sobin

Histological Typing of

Tumours of the Gallbladder and Extrahepatic Bile Ducts

2nd ed. 1991. XI, 77 pp. 80 figs. Softcover. ISBN 3-540-52838-5

K. Shanmugaratnam

Histological Typing of

Tumours of the Upper Respiratory Tract and Ear

In Collaboration with L. H. Sobin

2nd ed. 1991. Approx. 160 pp. 200 figs. Softcover. ISBN 3-540-53880-1

G. Seifert

Histological Typing of

Salivary Gland Tumours

In Collaboration with L. H. Sobin

2nd ed. 1991. XI, 112 pp. 130 figs. Softcover. ISBN 3-540-54031-8

I. R. H. Kramer, J. J. Pindborg, M. Shear

Histological Typing of

Odontogenic Tumours

2nd ed. 1991. Approx. 100 pp. 142 figs. Softcover. ISBN 3-540-54142-X

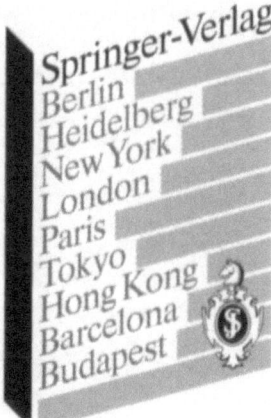

Springer-Verlag
Berlin
Heidelberg
New York
London
Paris
Tokyo
Hong Kong
Barcelona
Budapest

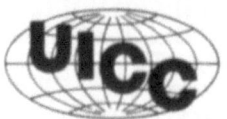 International
Union Against Cancer

B. Spiessl, O. H. Beahrs, P. Hermanek,
R. V. P. Hutter, O. Scheibe, L. H. Sobin,
G. Wagner (Eds.)

TNM Atlas

**Illustrated Guide to the TNM/pTNM
Classification of Malignant Tumours**

Illustrations by U. Kerl-Jentzsch, J. Kühn

3rd ed. 1989. Corr. reprint 1990. XIX, 343 pp.
452 figs. and an insert with summaries of the
T and N definitions by site.
Softcover. ISBN 3-540-17721-3

The TNM classification of malignant tumours
has the following objectives:
- to help the clinician determine the
  prognosis,
- to help the clinician in the planning
  of treatment,
- to assist in evaluating the results
  of treatment,
- to facilitate the exchange of information
  among treatment centres, and
- to contribute to the continuing investigation
  of human cancer.
The **TNM Atlas** is designed as an aid for the
practical application of the TNM classification
system. The corrected reprint includes the
latest FIGO changes in the classification for
corpus uteri and vulva carcinoma and a new
insert with summaries of the T and N definitions by site.

P. Hermanek, L. H. Sobin (Eds.)

TNM Classification
of Malignant Tumours

4th fully rev. ed. 1987. 2nd corr. reprint 1991.
XVIII, 197 pp. Softcover.
ISBN 3-540-17366-8

The TNM System is the most widely used
classification of the extent of growth and the
spread of cancer. Specific changes in the
fourth edition include:
- elimination of all differences between the
  AJCC (American Joint Committee on
  Cancer) and the UICC TNM classifications
  of head and neck tumours and lung
  tumours,
- revision of the T classifications of esopha-
  geal and gastric carcinomas based on
  Japanese studies,
- modification of the classification of colorec-
  tal tumours to provide direct congruence
  with the Dukes' classification and allow
  for a finer degree of subdivision,
- redrafting in collaboration with FIGO
  of the FIGO classification of gynecological
  tumours in the format of TNM, and
- addition of TNM classification for sites not
  previously covered in earlier
  UICC editions.

D. K. Hossfeld (Chairman), C. D. Sherman, R. R. Love,
F. X. Bosch (Eds.)

Manual of Clinical Oncology

5th ed. 1990. XIV, 391 pp. 88 figs. 69 tabs.
Softcover. ISBN 3-540-52769-9

The UICC **Manual of Clinical Oncology** has become a
basic textbook for all students and practitioners. It gives
concise, clear information on the concepts and underlying
principles which govern optimal cancer prevention,
diagnosis and treatment. The manual focuses intentionally
on basic aspects and does not go into details of therapy,
which are ever changing and controversial.
The fifth, fully revised edition has new chapters on carci-
nogenesis and prevention as well as many new tables and
figures. The text is easy to understand and covers the basic
and clinical biology of cancer in all its breadth.

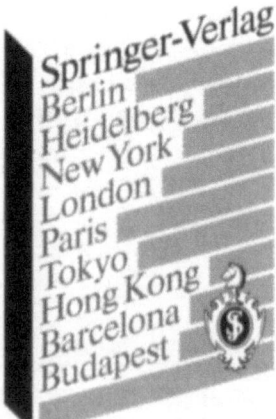

Springer-Verlag
Berlin
Heidelberg
New York
London
Paris
Tokyo
Hong Kong
Barcelona
Budapest